The ELECTROENCEPHALOGRAM
of the NORMAL CHILD

The ELECTROENCEPHALOGRAM of the NORMAL CHILD

By
ALBERTO FOIS, M.D.

Assistant and Docent of Pediatrics
University of Siena

Translated and edited by
NIELS L. LOW, M.D., F.A.A.P.

Assistant Professor of Neurology
Columbia University College of Physicians and Surgeons
New York

With Prefaces by
Professor Dr. Angelo Chieffi
and
Frederic A. Gibbs, M.D.

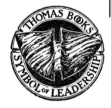

CHARLES C THOMAS • PUBLISHER

Springfield • Illinois • U.S.A.

CHARLES C THOMAS • PUBLISHER
Bannerstone House
301-327 East Lawrence Avenue, Springfield, Illinois, U.S.A.

© 1961, by CHARLES C THOMAS • PUBLISHER
Library of Congress Catalog Card Number: 60-15847

Printed in the United States of America

Italian edition dedicated to
Professor Dr. Angelo Chieffi

English edition dedicated to the memory of
Dr. Otto Low

The collection of tracings on which the publication of this volume is based has been made possible through the valuable cooperation of Dr. G. Franci and G. M. Ferri. The electroencephalograms were recorded at the Pediatric Clinic of the University of Siena, with a Galileo 8-channel console. The cost of publishing this material was borne in part by a grant from the National Research Council.

Preface

It is a pleasure to write this preface and to recommend this atlas by Dr. Alberto Fois, who has already made other valuable contributions to the electroencephalographic literature while working with the great expert in this field, Professor Dr. F. A. Gibbs in Chicago.

Those who are interested in this subject know with what skepticism the first electroencephalograms on children were received, and we all remember how analogous features in children with various disorders were interpreted by some as pathologic, by others as normal. Experience has shown that the latter have often been right; now we know how profound the differences are between EEGs of adults and those of children because of the slow maturation which is peculiar to the central nervous system compared to other body systems. These variations caused in the beginning some persons to assert that there was very little purpose in electroencephalographic investigation of infants because of the lack of cooperation from the youngest children and from those who could not cooperate for psychological reasons and because of the marked variability of the tracings in the different age groups. The most recent studies have justified not only the early enthusiasm but also the pessimism of the immediately following period.

A large amount of research has considerably increased our understanding of the special aspects of the EEGs of children and has allowed us to recognize with certainty if what we see in their records is normal or not. These results are possible today because of those who are active in this field and know how to master the technique and adhere to stringent criteria of interpretation and, therefore, can distinguish between brain waves from children of different ages and adults.

Dr. Fois' book has precisely this purpose, and I believe he succeeded perfectly; namely, to explain in a simple, clear form, and with detailed documentation both the basic technique for obtaining excellent records on the child and particular characteristics of the EEG from the first month through the fourteenth year. This knowledge, already in itself interesting, enriches the science of development of the central nervous system of children and, through this new method of investigation of the variations of bioelectrical potentials of the brain in different age groups, we are learning still more. Thorough comprehension of this material is indispensable to anyone who wants to work with abnormal electroencephalograms.

Therefore, I am expressing my best wishes that this book by Dr. Fois should meet with favor and approval of the reader. I also want to express in his and in my own name our gratitude to the National Research Council and the publishing firm "Omnia Medica" for their valuable contribution and the care they exercised in the production of this atlas.

ANGELO CHIEFFI

Preface To English Edition

The Italian edition of *L'Elettroencefalogramma del Bambino Normale* was so lucid, well illustrated and useful that it demanded an English translation. Dr. Fois, in collaboration with Dr. Niels L. Low, has produced an English edition which improves on the original.

Verbal description cannot convey the mass of detail that is needed for the diagnosis and precise interpretation of electroencephalograms. The written word can only underline certain aspects of the electroencephalogram and indicate its meaning. Accurate reading of such tracings requires experience with actual examples; this book helps to provide such experience.

The reduction of electroencephalograms to two-thirds their original size, which is used for the illustrations in the present volume, does not result in a loss of significant detail. The eye and brain are astonishingly competent at "enlarging" these reproductions so that they correspond in scale to unreduced recordings. Full scale reproduction, of course, has advantages but compactness also has advantages. Decreased cost and convenience of reference are strongly in favor of miniaturization. In this book a large series of tracings and many important facts have been compressed as far as visibility and readability would allow; it is little because it contains no fat.

Emphasis on the electroencephalograms of infants is advantageous. They differ from those of children and adults and they constitute a special problem; although electroencephalograms of adults and school children are abundant, teaching material on infants' electroencephalograms is scarce. This book performs an important service; it organizes and systematically presents examples of the characteristic electroencephalographic patterns encountered in infants, and it will add to general understanding and practical competence.

FREDERIC A. GIBBS, M.D.

Contents

List of Electroencephalograms

22.	8 months	Awake	45
23.	8 months	Drowsy	46
24.	8 months	Sleep	47
25.	8 months	Arousal	48
26.	9 months	Awake	49
27.	9 months	Drowsy	50
28.	9 months	Sleep	51
29.	9 months	Arousal	52
30.	10½ months	Awake	53
31.	10 months	Drowsy	54
32.	10 months	Arousal	55
33.	10½ months	Awake	56
34.	10½ months	Drowsy	57
35.	11 months	Awake	58
36.	11 months	Sleep	59
37.	11 months	Deep Sleep	60
38.	11 months	Arousal	61
39.	12 months	Awake	62
40.	12 months	Asleep	63
41.	12 months	Arousal	64
42.	21 months	Awake	65
43.	14 months	Drowsy	66
44.	16 months	Very light sleep	67
45.	16 months	Sleep	68
46.	16 months	Arousal	69
47.	2 years	Awake	70
48.	2 years	Drowsy	71

76.	9 years	Very light sleep	99
77.	9 years	Sleep	100
78.	9 years	Very deep sleep	101
79.	9 years	Arousal	102
80.	10 years	Awake	103
81.	10 years	Drowsy	104
82.	10 years	Sleep	105
83.	10 years	Deep sleep	106
84.	10 years	Arousal	107
85.	11 years	Awake	108
86.	11 years	Very light sleep	109
87.	11 years	Sleep	110
88.	11 years	Arousal	111
89.	12 years	Awake	112
90.	12 years	Light sleep	113
91.	12 years	Sleep	114
92.	12 years	Arousal	115
93.	13 years	Awake	116
94.	13 years	Drowsy	117
95.	13 years	Sleep	118
96.	13 years	Deeper sleep	119
97.	13 years	Arousal	120
98.	14 years	Awake	121
99.	14 years	Light sleep	122
100.	14 years	Deep sleep	123
101.	14 years	Arousal	124

The ELECTROENCEPHALOGRAM
of the NORMAL CHILD

ABBREVIATIONS

FS	Left Frontal
FD	Right Frontal
TS	Left Temporal
TD	Right Temporal
PS	Left Parietal
PD	Right Parietal
OS	Left Occipital
OD	Right Occipital

Introduction

The recording of electrical cerebral potentials had already become an indispensable tool of investigation in many instances although it is a relatively new field. Even since Berger published his remarkable investigations in 1929, much progress has been made, and electroencephalography has made such progress that it now is a very helpful additional test in neurological examination. Not only has this technique helped to define some diseases more clearly, but it has also increased our knowledge of the physiology of the central nervous system. Systemic examination of cerebral potentials has indeed made it possible to demonstrate electrical activity in intrauterine life (Lindsley 1942, Kennard 1942, Flexner 1949, Gibbs 1949) and changes with age which are characterized by increasing frequency in better organization until complete maturity of the electroencephalogram is reached by the age of thirty years. But even after this age changes occur into advanced age, at which time this evolution stops or even reverses. The different areas of the brain do not reach maturity at the same time. Grossman (1955) has shown different characteristic maturation of different brain areas. Additional striking differences are also observed between waking and sleep, induced by drugs, by hyperventilation, and between attention and relaxation. Generally speaking, there are numerous physiological and pathological factors which modify this already complex activity. Therefore, the expert electroencephalographer has to be familiar with the various features of the electroencephalogram with regard to the age of the patient, the state of waking, sleep and arousal, etc. Indeed, it is only the proper knowledge of the normal EEG and its variations which permits us to use this diagnostic aid safely.

For this reason, it is believed appropriate to present systematically as true as possible a number of tracings of normal children up to fourteen years of age in the waking state and physiologic sleep and arousal.

PHYSIOLOGY

It is known that all chemical and physical processes which take place in living cells produce electrical energy which can be recognized by changes in potential of the cell membrane. The potential produced by one single cell is very small, but when a larger group of cells functions in synchrony, the potential is proportionately higher and can well be recorded with suitable amplification. Recordings of the electrical potentials of the brain and heart are based on this principle. The EEG recorded through the intact skull, as it is usually done in routine clinical practice, can be considered the result of synchronous and rhythmic activity of groups of cortical neurons. These groups of neurons can also discharge with their own particular rhythm even when isolated from the rest of the brain. Spontaneous and rhythmical electrical activity can also be observed in the brain stem (Blake and Monnier, 1938; Ten-Cate and Koopman, 1940), in the cerebellum (Dow, 1938), and in the basal ganglia (Spiegel, 1937). Spontaneous cortical activity is relatively slower (Bremer, 1936).

It is conventional to call the input connections on each channel *Grid* 1 and *Grid* 2. Grid 1 is the input which when driven negative, with respect to the other, produces an upward deflection of the pen. In monopolar recordings connections are made from various areas over the cortex to Grid 1 on each channel; the reference electrode is connected to Grid 2. An upward deflection of the pen in the recording signifies negativity of the scalp electrode with respect to the reference electrode.

In general, the nearer the exploring (scalp) electrode is to a spike focus, the bigger (higher voltage), sharper, simpler, and more purely negative the spike discharge will be. When the spike focus is nearer to the common reference electrode than it is to the exploring electrodes a positive (downward) spike is registered in all channels. If the exploring electrode is moved farther and farther away from a spike focus, the amplitude (voltage) of the spike, as registered in the tracing, decreases and reverses its electrical sign, i.e., becomes positive instead of negative. This reversal was demonstrated experimentally by Curtis (1940), Dusser de Barenne, and McCulloch (1938).

During sleep, the cortical areas are more under the influence of the deep centers; in the cat under barbiturate anesthesia, the spontaneous activity which appears in the form of spindles with a frequency of 5 to 10 per second is under the influence of the thalamus. Recordings from the amygdala and the anterior commissure have shown a slow rhythm of 2 to 3 per second (Dempsey and Morison 1942). Moruzzi and Magoun (1949) have described a cortico-activating system in the reticular grey matter of the brain stem. This activating system exerts its influence by way of thalamic pathways. Lesions in the mesencephalic part of the system produce EEG changes which resemble those of normal sleep.

Changes of chemical constituents, especially of oxygen, carbon dioxide, glucose, sodium and potassium (Brazier, 1944; Bremer, 1936; Davis, 1943; Gibbs, 1940; Rubin, 1948; Gellhorn, 1942) modify cerebral electrical activity. Changes in the EEG can also be seen in metabolic diseases, such as phenylketonuria (Fois *et al.*, 1955; Low *et al.*, 1957) and other aberrations (Low, 1960). Reduction of oxygen and of glucose produce slowing of the electrical activity; reducing carbon dioxide will have the same effect. Slowing can also be produced by hypokalemia and hyponatremia (Chaptal, 1956). Hormones can also influence the EEG tracings (Faure, 1956).

INSTRUMENTATION

The electroencephalograph is an instrument which consists basically of an amplifying apparatus and a recording system. In its basic principle, it can be compared with an electrocardiograph; the lesser voltage of cerebral potentials makes great amplification necessary and, in addition, complexity of the brain makes it desirable to record from several areas simultaneously. Each separate amplifying unit with its recording unit is called a channel.

At least eight channels should be required of a modern clinical apparatus; instruments with sixteen and even more channels are now on the market. Eight channels are adequate for most clinical usage, in which that many cortical areas are recorded simultaneously. If necessary, two or more machines can be used at the same time. In most laboratories, a recording speed of 30 mm. per second is used although the instrument can be adjusted to speeds of 15 or 60 mm. per second.

All tracings which will be pictured in this book have been recorded at 30 mm. per second; this is a suitable standard to which visual memory can easily refer.

TECHNIQUE

The actual recording of the electroencephalogram does not present great difficulties; one can learn the basic technique by running a relatively small number of tracings. But it is necessary to run several hundreds of records to become an expert technician. Much more experience is needed to learn to interpret electroencephalograms in order to be able to recognize the various changes with age and physiological state. It is of utmost importance that whoever desires to interpret EEGs have adequate experience with both normal and abnormal records.

MONOPOLAR AND BIPOLAR RECORDING

In electroencephalography monopolar and bipolar recordings are being used. In the first instance, all electrodes are fastened to the skin of the intact skull and are related to one or two interconnected reference electrodes. In the second case, various areas of the surface are examined in comparison to each other, two at a time. Either method can give good results in the hands of the person who is experienced in that particular technique. One of the advantages of monopolar recordings is that it makes the interpretation of sleep records easier; this method is usually used in this laboratory. All EEGs presented in this atlas were done by monopolar technique.

APPLICATION OF ELECTRODES

According to our technique, the electrodes are applied symmetrically in pairs in the frontal, midtemporal, anterior temporal, central or parietal and occipital regions. When it is deemed advisable, additional electrodes may be applied. Reference electrodes are applied to the ear lobes; these are not necessarily inactive but are nevertheless very useful for good localization. In fact, when the ear lobe is active and therefore negative in relation to other points on the skull, these negative potentials will be transmitted through the common electrodes, as positive deflections in all surface electrodes except the one nearest the active ear. In such a situation, one can use the opposite ear alone as reference to avoid the spread to the skull leads. This is mainly the case in potentials arising from the anterior or midtemporal lobe. In this laboratory, we usually interconnect the two ear lobes in order to have a relatively inactive reference.

Reference electrodes over the sternum and the

spine have also been used but have not proven practical in clinical experience.

With many of the electroencephalographs on the market, one has to ground the patient to avoid an alternating current artifact. As a further precaution against artifact, resistance between skull and electrodes should be kept below 20,000 and between the two ear electrodes below 15,000 ohms.

ELECTRODES

The type of electrode used and the mode of application is also of importance for good recording. We use small silver disk electrodes which are connected to the apparatus by very thin insulated wires in a manner that permits the patient to move his head. These electrodes are fastened to the skull with cotton soaked with collodium, which is then dried rapidly with air from a hair-dryer or a compressed-air hose if the latter is available. After the recording, the electrodes are removed with acetone. In order to reduce skin resistance, it will sometimes be necessary to reduce scalp oil by washing with soap and water. With sufficient practice, one can apply 12 to 14 electrodes in 20 minutes. With good technique, a resistance between 5,000 and 20,000 ohms will be obtained. Between the electrodes and the skin a very small amount of bentonite paste is applied; we use the following formula:

Bentonite powder - 80 grams.
Calcium chloride - 80 grams.
Glycerin   - 30 ml.
Distilled water - q.s. to make a semiliquid paste.

With the technique employed by us, and the kind of electrode described, artifacts caused by displacement of electrodes and movement of patients can be practically eliminated. These electrodes can be made by the electroencephalographer or the technician himself, and they do not bother the patient and will not interfere with sleep when the conditions are otherwise suitable for it. Solder electrodes (60% tin and 40% lead) are also very good for electroencephalography; these have the advantages of costing very little. Many other kinds of electrodes are used in various other laboratories. The type described and used by us is superior to others regarding tolerability, adhesiveness, and true recording (Grass, 1948). Even if more time is required for our technique compared to some others, this disadvantage is more than compensated by the high quality of the records obtained. For the localization of electrical potentials originating in the basal ganglia, the use of pharyngeal and tympanic electrodes has been reported.

ENVIRONMENT

Especially when working with children, it is very important that the space is suitable both for the patient and the apparatus. It is desirable that the space for the patient is separate from the area where the technical equipment is kept so that the patient will not be frightened by the presence of the electroencephalograph. The space for the patient should be sound-proofed to facilitate spontaneous sleep, which is a very useful activation method, and which will avoid much artifact which can be very disturbing to infants and young children. The walls of the room also should be painted in colors that are as pleasant as possible to the subject. If alternating current causes artifacts, it may be necessary to equip the room with a grounded metal screen or cage which should be covered with a material that can be fitted with acoustic tiling; it is important that the patient not be frightened by a visible enclosure. The lights and wiring in the laboratory also have to be suitably screened and the power for the electroencephalo-

graph should come preferably from a separate conduit which does not feed other equipment, especially diathermy or x-ray.

AIDS FOR OBTAINING GOOD RECORDINGS

Following the above recommendations is usually sufficient to obtain spontaneous sleep in a high percentage of patients, if they are not exceptionally apprehensive. Recording during waking as well as in the various stages of sleep is essential because this physiological state has proven to be a good activator for electroencephalographic abnormalities, especially in epilepsy (Gibbs, 1952; Kellaway, 1952). A tracing obtained only while the patient is awake cannot be regarded as complete. When the examiner wants to be certain of obtaining sleep in a patient, it is necessary that the patient sleep less than usually the night previous to the examination. In infants it is usually sufficient to perform the test in early afternoon, avoiding a morning nap. Feeding the patient will considerably facilitate sleep; in a little older child, limiting the preceding night's sleep from three to six hours is helpful. In the case of very apprehensive children it is sometimes permissible to allow the mother to remain in the room.

METHOD OF RECORDING

Once the electrodes have been applied and the resistance between them has been found to not exceed 20,000 ohms, the recording can be performed while the patient is awake, during sleep and arousal. In the beginning and following the examination, the machine has to be calibrated. We prefer to use an amplification which registers 7 mm./50 microvolts; at times it is preferable to use a 5 mm/microvolt deflection in children. If, after a reasonable time, the patient has not fallen asleep and is restless, one can administer a fast-acting barbiturate, such as Seconal (30 to 200 mg, depending on the patient's age.) One must remember, however, that such a drug may cause fast activity of 10 to 25 cycles per second.

If the patient can cooperate sufficiently, he should hyperventilate for two to three minutes after arousal. The response will vary considerably with age (Brill, 1941; Gibbs, 1943); the slowing which is obtained in a child is much more marked than in an adult. This activation method has in our experience been of help only in petit mal in which an increase of the typical generalized 3 per second spike and wave pattern is produced. On the other hand, drowsiness will also be an excellent activator in this condition.

OTHER PROCEDURES OF ACTIVATION

Among other activating methods, photostimulation (Gastaut, 1948) is indicated mainly when photogenic or myoclonus epilepsy is suspected; it is not used much in our laboratory. We rarely employ activation with Metrazol (Cook, 1938; Davis, 1939; Rubin, 1939) although other investigators use it more frequently. According to the work of Moore and Kellaway (1955), abnormal potentials elicited by this method are only of significance when they are focal; when generalized discharges are produced in this manner, they are not indicative of epilepsy because of the variability of individual sensitivity to Metrazol even in normal people. For that reason, it is difficult to distinguish between convulsive activity due to Metrazol and true epilepsy. Acoustic stimulation (Arellano, 1950) and apnea (Silverman, 1956) are more of theoretical than of practical importance.

PERSONNEL

The application of electrodes and the recording can be carried out by the technician who has some knowledge of electrical physiology and has a fair ability of recognizing normal and abnormal electroencephalograms. It is not necessary, therefore, that a physician perform the task, but in order to obtain true interpretation of the records understanding of clinical correlation is essential. One has to have specific and thorough knowledge of the art and science of electroencephalography in order to avoid errors in interpretation.

GENERAL CHARACTERISTICS
OF THE NORMAL ENCEPHALOGRAM

For a detailed description and classification of the various types of brain waves, one should refer to manuals on this subject (Gibbs, 1950; Hill, 1950; Cobb, 1950; Gozzano, 1951) and many other publications regarding children (Bernhard, 1939; Bickford, 1955; Billie, 1955; DeToni, 1952; Dreyfus Brisac, 1955; Drohcki, 1938; Garsche, 1951-1953; Gibbs, 1944-1949; Gollnitz, 1952; Harguindegny, 1955; Hughes, 1948; Lombroso, 1951; Mozziconacci, 1947; Schultz, 1951; Shimoda, 1954; Smith, 1937; Smith, 1938; Soureau, 1950; Walter, 1949).

GENERAL CHARACTERISTICS
OF THE EEG IN WAKING

In general, one can say that the EEG consists of waves of various frequencies, forms and voltages. According to frequency, these waves may be classified into alpha (8 to 13 per second), teta (4 to 7 per second), delta (less than 4 per second), and beta (more than 13 per second). This classification is not followed by all investigators, who often prefer simply to indicate a frequency per second. The alpha rhythm is not present in the first year of life; it is best developed in the occipital area; it disappears with attention and the opening of the eyes. In small children and during sleep, slow frequencies predominate, but a small amount of fast activity can be seen even in the first year of life. Serial examinations of the same patients (Lindsley 1936) or of different patients in different age groups show that brain waves increase from slower to faster activity with age. *Above all, one must remember that the tracings through the first year of life show considerable individual variation and one can call abnormal only changes in rhythm which are very obviously different.*

GENERAL CHARACTERISTICS
OF THE EEG IN SPONTANEOUS SLEEP

The typical sleep EEG deserves particular attention. The brain waves in that state are variable; they are related to different stages of sleep (drowsiness, light and deep sleep, and arousal), to the age of the patient, and to the area of the brain examined

(Barnes, 1946; Blake, 1939; Davis, 1937; Gibbs, 1950; Hughes, 1948; Neckerocheff, 1950; Smith, 1938).

During drowsiness the dominant activity of an infant is slow and paroxysmal and an inexperienced observer might confuse this with a convulsive pattern, while in an adult only some flattening of the waves would be seen. During light sleep there appears a characteristic pattern which has been termed "humps" by Gibbs. Morphologically similar waves have been called K complexes (Davis, 1939); but these terms are not synonymous because the K complexes are paroxysmal changes in the parietal area caused by acustic stimuli in sleep. We prefer the term humps; they appear as slow, biphasic waves with a duration of ⅓ to ⅛ second. They are best seen in the parietal leads and are more frequent in older children.

Drowsiness is followed by light sleep; the characteristic feature of that stage is "spindles"; the spindles are best seen in parietal and frontal leads and have their name because they consist of sinusoidal waves with a waxing and waning amplitude. The duration of each spindle formation varies from 1 to 3 seconds; the voltage tends to vary with age,

being higher in older children. The frequency of spindles varies between 14 and 8 to 10 per second. Fourteen per second spindles are characteristic of light sleep and they first appear in parietal leads between three and nine months of age and are always symmetrical after 12 months of age. Twelve per second spindles are commonly seen in the frontal area in somewhat deeper sleep. Eight to 10 per second spindles may also be seen; they are more diffuse and are synchronous. In this phase of sleep, the basic activity consists of irregular, slow 6 per second waves of low voltage. Humps may still be present.

In deep sleep, the basic frequency is diffusely very slow with frequencies from 0.5 to 3 per second, with faster waves superimposed.

On arousal, different patterns are seen which also vary with the age of the child. In the newborn period, the transition from sleep to waking is not clearly marked, but is usually recognized by muscle artifacts. Later, a few slow waves appear which in the first few years of life last for several minutes and are similar to the pattern of drowsiness. These waves diminish in amplitude and increase in frequency until the normal waking state is reached.

The tracings presented in this volume were obtained from normal children. They represent patterns which are most commonly found in each respective age group. As mentioned before, they were all obtained with a standard technique in order to facilitate comparing them according to age. In all instances, the monopolar method with the interconnected ear lobes for reference were used with an amplification that gives a deflection of 7 mm/50 microvolts. Therefore, very high waves will sometimes deflect the pens to their maximal excursion. We do not use filters because they modify the form of the tracing. They are always recorded at a constant speed of 30 mm/second. In order to conserve space, the tables in this book are reproduced on a smaller scale with a dimension of 20 x 14 cm. instead of 30 x 20 cm. of the original records; however, the size of the reproduction is adequate to see all details.

TYPICAL FINDINGS
One Month to Three Months

Because of incomplete maturation of the brain and the relative inactivity of the cortex in this period of infancy, the differences between waking and sleep and among the different areas of the brain are less marked at this time than later. The electrical activity of the cortex during waking is probably entirely under the control of deeper centers in this period. This is apparently the reason that in our experience it is difficult to recognize focal abnormalities while diffuse changes can be seen.

The basic waking activity during the first few days of life is first recognized in the parietal area and consists of irregular, low voltage 3 to 5 per second waves with superimposed 6 to 9 per second activity; rarely, faster waves are seen. With increasing age, the voltage increases, and towards three months a distinct pattern tends to develop. Opening and closing of the eye does not cause changes in the waves in the frontal area that are seen at a later age.

At the end of this period, sleep produces a clear change; it is best seen in parietal and occipital leads when the rhythm becomes slower and the voltage higher. When sleep is of the proper depth, one can find some 10 to 15 per second spindles in the parieto-occipital area already during the first few weeks. But these are not fully developed in groups yet, as in later months, and are of lower voltage, and are relatively infrequent. During the second and third months, they acquire the typical morphology and occur more frequently. During the early months, the spindles are asynchronous, that is, they do not occur on the right and left side simultaneously; the age in which they become synchronous varies considerably but is usually reached at the end of the first year, occasionally during the second year.

Changes of deep sleep are not often obtained at this age but when present are characterized by further slowing and increase of amplitude. Arousal does not cause a typical pattern but it is principally recognized by the appearance of muscle artifact; the paroxysmal slowing in tracings of older children is not yet seen. Only a hint of such a pattern can be distinguished in the three-months old baby.

The asynchrony which can be seen between homonymous brain areas must be kept in mind at all times; also, the individual differences in focal and generalized slowing have to be judged with great care.

Four Months to One Year

This is a period in which the EEG undergoes the changes which give it by the end of the first year the fundamental characteristics of the first decade. A gradual increase of waking rhythm is seen, and also some of the sleep frequencies.

The waking rhythm at first is between 4 and 7 per second in a four-months old child and the tracing appears more organized in the central leads. A tendency to an increase of voltage and frequency is seen parallelling increasing age, and at the end of the year the basic frequency is 6 to 8 per second, best seen in the occipital area. But individual variations exist in this age group also. Until six months of age, asynchrony and asymmetry are still normal while awake but with increasing age these features acquire significance and by one year they have to be regarded as abnormal.

Sleep induces clear changes in activity; drowsiness causes general slowing and an increase of voltage, most marked in the parietal leads. The difference between drowsiness and light sleep may not be clearly present until after six months. In this first stage of sleep some paroxysmal slowing may be seen, but it becomes more evident after the first year. In this age, humps are first noted; they are diphasic and resemble high voltage spikes in the parietal leads, occasionally also in other areas; their occurrence increases with age. In the next stage of sleep, spindles are seen, least evident in the younger patients. They can be easily recognized and they have a frequency of 13 to 15 per second and are best seen in the parietal, less in the frontal leads. The basic pattern consists of irregular 3 to 6 per second waves with superimposed low voltage fast activity. Asynchrony may still be present, especially in the parietal area, and does not yet indicate abnormality. A high percentage of children will also show fast 18 to 22 per second activity while awake and in all stages of sleep except deep sleep.

Deep sleep is recognized by further slowing and irregular high waves without humps and spindles.

Arousal becomes differentiated with increase in age from four months to one year. With increase in age, paroxysmal synchronous slowing with high voltage sinusoidal waves appears in all leads; they have a frequency of 2 to 4 per second. The duration of this stage varies from one patient to another but a pattern is clearly paroxysmal in some cases; the changes may be more gradual, appoaching the waking EEG. After arousal some occipital slowing may persist which is not pathological.

The Second and Third Years

The EEG in this age group displays more clearly the characteristics first found at the end of the first year. The basic waking rhythm contains more fast activity but the dominant frequency is 6 to 8 per second, best developed in the parietal and occipital leads. Four to 6 per second waves still occur.

Paroxysmal slowing during drowsiness is particularly marked in this period. These high voltage sinusoidal waves have a frequency of about 3 per second and are seen in all leads. The slowing has a tendency to occur in runs but more often it has a tendency to continue for a duration of up to one minute.

In light sleep, humps are always present; they are now synchronous, of high voltage, and best seen in the parietal area. First they occur alone but later with spindles. The latter are now of typical appearance, are synchronous, and also are most marked in the central leads. Their frequency varies from 12 to 15 per second and they may be seen in occipital, and more frequently in frontal leads. Frequently in the first stage of sleep, fast rhythms of the type described in infants are seen. They disappear in deeper sleep. The characteristics of deep sleep are similar to those in younger children.

Arousal has a strong resemblance to drowsiness; in fact, paroxysmal slowing of varying length is practically always present. After awakening slowing in the occipital area is seen for some time.

The Fourth and Fifth Years

During waking a further increase of frequency is seen and is more uniform in the record. On the other hand, there are no fundamental differences between brain waves in children of this age group compared with those two years old. Although some 8 to 10 per second frequencies occur, basic activity still consists of 8 per second waves and is best developed in the occipital leads. Mixed with these frequencies are also some 4 to 5 per second rhythms. The voltage is now higher than it was in younger children and the waves are synchronous. A definite asymmetry is now abnormal. Only in the temporal lobes can minor differences be regarded as physiological. Drowsiness is characterized by flattening of the record and by the occurrence of some paroxysmal 3 per second slowing of short duration; the findings described in the second year of life can also be noted

in this age. Slowing, however, is of shorter duration now and is seen as runs of 3 per second waves, mainly in the frontal and parietal areas. Some notching of the waves is sometimes seen and, therefore, they have been erroneously diagnosed as petit mal discharges. This finding may be present through the eighth year.

In light sleep, high voltage becomes frequent, always best seen in the parietal leads and asynchronous spindles are also higher than previously and their frequency varies from 12 to 15 per second.

In deep sleep, the EEG looks essentially the same as it did in younger children. Arousal resembles drowsiness, and again the paroxysmal slowing in this age is of shorter duration than in the two-year age group.

From the Fifth to the Seventh Year

The waking EEG at rest has a basic occipital rhythm of 7 to 9 per second but there is also some slower 5 to 6 per second and some faster 10 to 12 per second activity. The waves are symmetrical, and opening of the eyes causes a marked flattening of the record.

Paroxysmal slowing can still be found in drowsiness but often a flattening is observed together with some irregular fast activity.

In light sleep humps appear. They attain the highest voltage in this age group, may occur in groups, and are bilaterally synchronous. Although they are mainly a characteristic feature of the parietal area, they can sometimes be recorded from all leads. High voltage spindles start always immediately after the first humps. Their frequency varies somewhat with the depth of sleep, being slower as sleep deepens. First they have a frequency of 13 to 15 per second with parieto-occipital predominance but they may be seen in other leads, too. In the frontal region, there may be independent 11 to 12 per second spindles which may be asynchronous. In later stages of sleep, spindles may slow to 9 to 10 per second with very high voltage, mainly in the frontal area, but occasionally also seen in other leads. The features just described are characteristic of this age.

Deep sleep has no specific form but is characterized by irregular slow activity with some faster waves superimposed.

On awakening some paroxysmal slowing of brief duration may be seen but marked variations without pathological significance may occur. In a small percentage of patients, a sudden transition from sleep to waking without an arousal pattern occurs.

From the Eighth to the Tenth Year

At this age there is a tendency for a lower voltage compared to younger children.

The dominant waking frequency is from 8 to 12 per second; in general, the frequencies are higher when the voltage is lower. A certain amount of 6 to 7 per second activity is still seen. A basic rhythm is best seen in the occipital area. In that area patterns may occur which superficially resemble spikes and waves. In doubtful cases, these features can be recognized as not abnormal because they disappear in sleep, while true seizure discharges would become more apparent in that state.

Drowsiness causes flattening of the waves. In this age group, paroxysmal slowing is not regularly present and, when present, it looks different from the slowing in younger children; it appears in the form of runs of 5 to 6 per second activity of a few seconds duration.

Humps are always present in light sleep but their voltage is lower than described in previous paragraphs. They are very frequent with a clear parietal localization and are rarely seen in other leads. If sleep is a little deeper, spindles will also always appear; they, too, are of lower voltage now. The spindles have a frequency of 14 per second, are seen in the parietal leads, while 12 per second spindles may be recorded from the frontal area. Rarely, 10 per second spindles are seen at this age.

Nothing which is specific for this age group is seen in deep sleep.

In arousal, there is regularly a tendency for paroxysmal slowing. But beyond the seventh year this slowing is of shorter duration with a frequency of 5 to 7 per second.

From the Eleventh to the Fourteenth Year

The tracing tends to show the characteristic features of an adult EEG. A further tendency to reduction of voltage takes place which becomes more marked with increasing age, while paroxysmal slowing, normal in younger age groups, becomes rare. During waking, the normal frequency is 8 to 10 per second, but 13 to 14 per second activity is not uncommon. Faster waves should be regarded as being outside the normal range. Although the voltage is usually not very high, it occasionally is higher than 100 microvolts. Alpha rhythm is best developed in occipital leads; it is clearly affected by opening of the eyes and in state of relaxation.

Drowsiness causes flattening of the record; sinusoidal waves of medium voltage in the frontal leads are characteristic in this age. They have a frequency of 5 to 7 per second and the voltage is rarely above 100 microvolts and lasts approximately 3 to 4 per second. This slowing is not present in all subjects, but is normal when it occurs.

Paroxysmal slowing can be seen in some children, but is then only of short duration with a frequency of 4 to 7 per second and only slightly increased voltage. Often only the previously described flattening of the record is seen; but a few patients may have a small amount of low voltage 15 to 18 per second activity.

In light sleep, humps occur regularly; their amplitude is moderately high with a maximum voltage of 200 microvolts; they occur characteristically in the parietal area but may also be seen in other leads. The humps are less frequent than they were in younger children. The amplitude of spindles is also lower and their frequency is highest in the early stages of sleep and almost entirely limited to the parietal area. Twelve per second spindles occur in somewhat deeper sleep and are more pronounced in the frontal leads although they may be diffuse; some asynchrony can be seen in normal subjects. These frontal spindles may end with a slow after-discharge at this age and, therefore, can be confused with spike and wave discharges by the inexperienced observer.

We have already seen that there is very little difference between the age groups in deep sleep but extreme slowing is uncommon past ten years of age.

Also, in arousal, marked slowing is usually absent; in general, the transition from sleep to wakening is rather sudden. If paroxysmal slowing is present it is often limited to the frontal area and the frequency does not go below 4 per second. In fact, it is usually from 5 to 7 per second without much increase in voltage.

In addition to supplying the data for the interpretation of electroencephalograms of children, the following figures illustrate the dynamic development of the brain in early life.

Through the study of EEGs, we observe one facet of the changes which the brain undergoes in the process of maturation and aging, processes which are more complex in the brain than in most other organs. These observations make the hypothesis likely that the biochemical processes change from childhood to the adult of thirty or seventy years. These relationships, however, are still a subject of speculation.

It would certainly be of great importance if one day someone could correlate electrical activity of the neurons with their cellular metabolism. When technical equipment can be built to measure and record all of these metabolic processes, it will still be less perfect than the human brain which designed it.

References

ARELLANO, A. P., SCHWAB, R. S., and CASBY, I. V.: Sonic activation. *Electroencephalog. & Clin. Neurophysiol.*, 2:215, 1950.

BARNES, T. C., RUTH, H. S., and HULTZMAN, E. K.: Electroencephalography of infants under pentothal anesthesia. *Federation Proc.*, 5:6, 1946.

BERGER, H.: Ueber das Elektrenzephalogram des Menschen. *Arch. Psychiat.*, 87:527, 1929.

BARNHARD, C. G., and SKOGLUND, C. R.: Alpha frequency of human brain potentials as function of age. *Scandinav. Arch. Physiol.*, 82:178, 1939.

BICKFORD, R. C., KEITH, H. M.: Electroencephalography in Pediatrics. *Quart. Rev. Pediat.*, 10:69, 1955.

BILLE, S., and BRANOTTI, S.: The normal E.E.G. in infants and small children. *Acta. paediat.*, Suppl 44:103, 1955.

BLAKE, H., and MONNIER, M.: Potentials from the medulla of the cat. *Am. J. Physiol.*, 123:17, 1938.

BLAKE, H.: Brain potential and depth of sleep. *Am. J. Physiol.*, 119:273, 1937.

BLAKE, H., and GERARD, R. W.: Brain potentials during sleep. *Am. J. Physiol.*, 119:692, 1937.

BLAKE, H., GERARD, R. W., and KLEITMAN, N.: Factors influencing brain potentials during sleep. *J. Neurophysiol.*, 2:48, 1939.

BRAZIER, M. A. B., FINESINGER, J. E., and SCHWAB, R. S.: Characteristics of the normal electroencephalogram. II. The effect of varying blood sugar levels on the occipital cortical potentials in adults during quiet breathing. *J. Clin. Investigation*, 23:313, 1944.

BREMER, F., and THOMAS, J.: Action de l'anoxémie, de l'hypercapnie et de l'acapnie sur l'activité électrique du cortex cérébral. *Compt. rend, Soc. de Biol.*, 123:1256, 1936.

BREMER, F.: Activité électrique du cortex cérébral dans les états de sommeil et de veille chez le chat. *Compt. Rend. Soc. de Biol.*, 122:353, 1936.

BRILL, N. W., and SEIDEMANN, H.: Electroencephalogram of normal children; effect of hyperventilation. *Am. J. Psychiat.*, 98:250, 1941.

CHAPTAL, J., *et al.*: Rôle de l'encéphalose métabolique au cours des atteintes méningo-encéphalitiques de l'enfance. *Pédiatrie*, 11:687, 897, 1956.

COHN, R.: *Clinical Electroencephalography*. New York, McGraw-Hill Book Company, 1950.

COOK, L. C., and WALTER, W. F.: The electroencephalogram in convulsions induced by cardiazol. *J. Neurol. &*

Psychiat., 1:180, 1938.

CURTIS, H. J.: Intercortical connections of corpus callosum as indicated by evoked potentials. *J. Neurophysiol., 3*:407, 1940.

DARROW, C. W.: Convenient electroencephalographic electrode. *Proc. Soc. Exper. Biol. & Med., 45*:301, 1940.

DAVIS, H., DAVIS, P. A., LOOMIS, A. L., and HARVEY, E. N.: Electrical responses of the human brain to auditory stimulation during sleep. *J. Neurophysiol. 1*:413, 1939.

DAVIS, H., DAVIS, P. A., LOOMIS, A. L., HARVEY, E. N., and HOBART, G.: Changes in human brain potentials during the onset of sleep. *Science, 86*:448, 1937.

DAVIS, H., DAVIS, P. A., LOOMIS, A. L., HARVEY, E. N., and HOBART, G.: Human brain potentials during the onset of sleep. *J. Neurophysiol., 1*:24, 1938.

DAVIS, P. A.: The electrical response of the human brain to auditory stimuli. *Am. J. Physiol., 126*:475, 1939.

DAVIS, P. A.: Effect on the electroencephalogram of changing blood sugar level. *Arch. Neurol. & Psychiat., 49*:186, 1943.

DAVIS, P. A., and SULZBACH, W.: Changes in electroencephalogram during metrazol therapy. *Tr. Am. Neurol. Acad., 65*:144, 1939.

DEMPSEY, E. W., and MORISON, R. S.: The production of rhythmically recurrent cortical potentials after localized thalamic stimulation. *Am. J. Physiol., 135*:243, 1942.

DE TONI, G.: La nostra esperienza in 350 esami EEG eseguiti nell'eta età infantile. *Minerva pediat., 43*:22, 1952.

DOW, R. S.: The electrical activity of the cerebellum and its functional significance. *J. Physiol., 94*:67, 1938.

DREYFUS-BRISAC, C., SAMSON, D., and FISCHGOLD, H.: Technique de l'enregistrement EEG du prématuré et du nouveau-né. *Electroencephalog. & Clin. Neurophysiol., 7*:429, 1955.

DROHOCKI, Z.: Les manifestions électriques spontanées du cerveau à l'état de veille. *Compt. rend. Soc. de Biol., 130*:99, 1938.

DUSSER DE BARENNE, J. G., McCULLOGH, W. S.: The direct functional interrelation of sensory cortex and optic thalamus. *J. Neurophysiol., 1*:176, 1938.

FAURE, J.: A comparison of the EEG with hormonal changes in female patients. *Electroencephalop. & Clin. Neurophysiol., 8*:172, 1956.

FLEXNER, L. B.: Studies on the development of the cortex of the brain. *Science, 110*:551, 1949.

FOIS, A., ROSENBERG, C., and GIBBS, F. A.: The EEG in phenylpyruvic oligophrenia. *Electroencephalog. & Clin. Neurophysiol., 7*:569, 1955.

GARSCHE, R.: Grundzüge des normalen Elektroencephalogram im Kindesalter. *Klin. Wchnschr., 118*:31, 1953.

GARSCHE, R., and DLUGOSCH, G.: Uber die klinische Bedeutung der Electroenzephalographie im Kindesalter. *Arch. Kinderheilk., 142*:65, 1951.

GASTAUT, H.: Sur un mode nouveau d'entraînement des rythmes corticaux par des stimulations photo-acoustiques intermittentes synchronisées. *Compt. Rend. Soc. Biol., 142*:351, 1948.

GELLHORN, E., and KESSLER, M.: Effect of hypoglycemia on electroencephalogram at varying degrees of oxygenation of blood. *Am. J. Physiol., 136*:1, 1942.

GIBBS, F. A.: Electrical activity of the brain. *Ann. Rev. Physiol., 7*:427, 1945.

GIBBS, F. A., and GIBBS, E. L.: Electroencephalographic changes with age in adolescent and adult control subjects. *Tr. Am. Neurol. A., 70*:154, 1944.

GIBBS, F. A., GIBBS, E. L., and LENNOX, W. G.: Electroencephalographic response to overventilation and its relation to age. *J. Pediat., 23*:497, 1943.

GIBBS, F. A., and GIBBS, E. L.: Atlas of Electroencephalography. Addison Wesley Press, Cambridge, Massachusetts, I, II, 1950, 1952.

GIBBS, F. A., and KNOTT, J. R.: Growth of the electrical activity of the cortex. *Electroencephalog. & Clin. Neurophysiol., 1*:223, 1949.

GIBBS, F. A., WILLIAMS, D., and GIBBS, E. L.: Modification of the cortical frequency spectrum by changes in CO_2 blood sugar and O_2. *J. Neurophysiol., 3*:49, 1940.

GIBBS, F. A., and LOW, N. L.: *Pediatric Clinics of North America.* Philadelphia, W. B. Saunders, February, 1955.

GÖLLNITZ, G.: Ueber das normale Encephalogram im Kindesalter. *Nervenarzt, 23*:466, 1952.

GOZZANO, R.: Ricerche sui fenomeni elettrici della corteccia cerebrale. *Riv. di neurol., 8*:212, 1935.

GOZZANO, R., and COLOMBATI, S.: *Compendio di Elettroencefalografia Clinica.* Rosenberg & Sellier, Torino, 1951.

GOZZANO, R.: L'attivita elettrica del cervello. *Rassegna Med., 43*:5, 1941.

GRASS, A. M.: Electrical characteristics of some types of electrodes. Reported at the meeting of Central Association of Electroencephalographers, April, 1948.

GROSSMAN, C.: Electro-ontogenesis of cerebral activity. *A.M.A. Arch. Neurol., & Psychiat., 74*:186, 1955.

HARGUINDEGNY, E., and IMBRIANO, A. E.: La electroencefalografia en el recien nacido normal, de parto normal. *Semana med., 106*:535, 1955.

HILL, N. D., and PARR, G.: *Electroencephalography.* London, McDonald & Company, 1950.

HUGHES, J. G.: EEG of the newborn (abnormal EEG of neonate). *Am. J. Dis. Child., 76*:634, 1948.

HUGHES, J. G., EHEMANN, B., and BROWN, V. A.: EEG of the newborn; studies on normal, full term infants while awake and while drowsy. *Am. J. Dis. Child., 77*:310, 1949.

HUGHES, J. G. *et al.*: EEG of the newborn; studies on normal, full term, sleeping infants. *Am. J. Dis. Child., 76*:503, 1948.

KELLAWAY, P., and Fox, B. J.: Electroencephalographic diagnosis of cerebral pathology in infants during sleep. I. Rationale, technique, and the characteristics of normal sleep in infants. *J. Pediat., 51*:262, 1952.

KENNARD, M. A., and NIMS, L. F.: Changes in normal electroencephalogram of Macaca Mulatta with growth. *J. Neurophysiol., 5*:325, 1942.

KIRSCHOFF, H. W., and FRÖLICH, B.: Elektroencephalographische Untersuchungen über den Schlaf des Säuglings. *Arch. Psychiat., 148*:341, 1952.

LINDSLEY, D. B.: Heart and brain potentials of human fetuses in utero. *Am. J. Physiol., 55*:412, 1942.

LINDSLEY, D. B.: Brain potentials in children and adults. *Science, 84*:354, 1956.

LENNOX, M. A., and LENNOX, W. G.: Electrical activity of the brain. *Ann. Rev. Physiol., 9*:507, 1947.

LOMBROSO, C., and GROSSI-BIANCHI, N. L.: Variazioni dello EEG nei primi 5 anni di vita. *Riv. Ped., 3*:120, 1951.

LOW, N. L., BOSMA, J. F., and ARMSTRONG, M. D.: Studies on Phenylketonuria. VI. EEG studies in phenylketonuria. *A.M.A. Arch. Neurol. Psychiat., 77*:359, 1957.

LOW, N. L.: Infantile spasms. Pediatric Clinics of North America. Philadelphia, W. B. Saunders, May, 1960.

MOORE, F. J., and KELLAWAY, P.: Metrazol activation as a diagnostic adjunct in electroencephalography. *A.M.A. Arch. Neurol. Psychiat., 73*:356, 1955.

MORUZZI, G., and MAGOUN, H. W.: Brain stem reticular formation and activation of the EEG. *Electroencephalog. & Clin. Neurophysiol., 1*:455, 1949.

MORUZZI, G., and MAGOUN, H. W.: Influence of bulboreticular stimulation upon electrical activity of cerebral cortex. *Federation Proc., 8*:113, 1949.

MOZZICONACCI, P., and LERIQUE, R.: L'EEG de l'enfant normal et son interprétation. *Nourrisson, 44*:35, 1947.

NEKHOROCHEFF, M. I.: L'EEG du sommeil chez l'enfant. *Revue neurol., 82*:487, 1950.

NEKHOROCHEFF, M. I.: L'EEG dans le sommeil spontané et le sommeil provoqué chez l'enfant. *Rev. neurol., 83*:575, 1950.

RUBIN, M. A., HOFF, H. E., WINKLER, A. W., and SMITH, K. O.: Intravenous potassium calcium and magnesium and the cortical electrogram of the cat. *J. Neurophysiol., 6*:23, 1948.

RUBIN, M. A., and TURNER, E.: Blood sugar level and influence of hyperventilation on slow activity in electroencephalogram. *Proc. Soc. Exper. Biol. & Med., 50*:270, 1942.

RUBIN, M. A., and WALL, C.: Brain potential changes in man induced by metrazol. *J. Neurol. Psychiat., 2*:107, 1939.

SCHULTZ, E., and DÜLLER, H. W.: Das kindliche Elektrenzephalogramm. *Klin. Wchnsch., 29*:20, 1951.

SHIMODA, Y., HANAZONO, N., KOIZUMI, A., et al.: EEG

changes and age factor. II. The frequency analysis, topographical abnormality and paroxysmal discharges of the EEG of normal children from 4 to 15 years of age. *Folia Psychiat. et Neurol. Japonica, 8*:202, 1954.

SILVERMAN, D. A.: Comparison of hyperventilation and apnea activation of the EEG. *Electroencephalog. & Clin. Neurophysiol., 8*:41, 1956.

SMITH, J. R.: Electroencephalogram during infancy and childhood. *Proc. Soc. Exper. Biol. & Med., 36*:384, 1937.

SMITH, J. R.: The electroencephalogram during normal infancy and childhood. I. Rhythmic activities present in the neonate and their subsequent development. *J. Gen. Psychol., 53*:431, 1938.

SMITH, J. R.: The electroencephalogram during normal infancy and childhood. II. The nature of the growth of the alpha waves. *J. Gen. Psychol., 53*:455, 1938.

SMITH, J. R.: The electroencephalogram during normal infancy and childhood. III. Preliminary observations on the pattern sequence during sleep. *J. Gen. Psychol., 53*:471, 1938.

SMITH, J. R.: The frequency growth of the human alpha rhythms during normal infancy and childhood. *J. Psychol., 11*:177, 1941.

SOUREAU, M. *et al.*: L'EEG du nouveau-né normal et pathologique. *Electroencephalog. & Clin. Neurophysiol., 2*:113, 1950.

SPIEGEL, C. A.: Comparative study of the thalamic cerebral and cerebellar potentials. *Am. J. Physiol., 118*:569, 1897.

STRAUSS, H., and RAHM, W. E., Jr.: Reactions of the electroencephalogram to metrazol injections. *Proc. Soc. Exper. Biol. & Med., 40*:1, 1939.

TEN CATE, J., and WIGGERS, K.: On the occurrence of slow waves in the electrocerebellogram. *Arch. Nederl. de Physiol., 26*:423, 1942.

TEN CATE, J., and WALTER, W. G.: Note on the electroencephalography of the brain stem and cerebellum of cats. *Arch. Nederl. de Physiol., 25*:51, 1940.

WALTER, W. G., DOVEY, V. J., and SHIPTON, H.: Analysis of the electrical responses of human cortex to photic stimulation. *Nature, 158*:540, 1946.

WALTER, W. G., and WALTER, V. J.: The electrical activity of the brain. *Ann. Rev. Physiol., 11*:199, 1949.

FIGURE 1. — *One month, awake.*

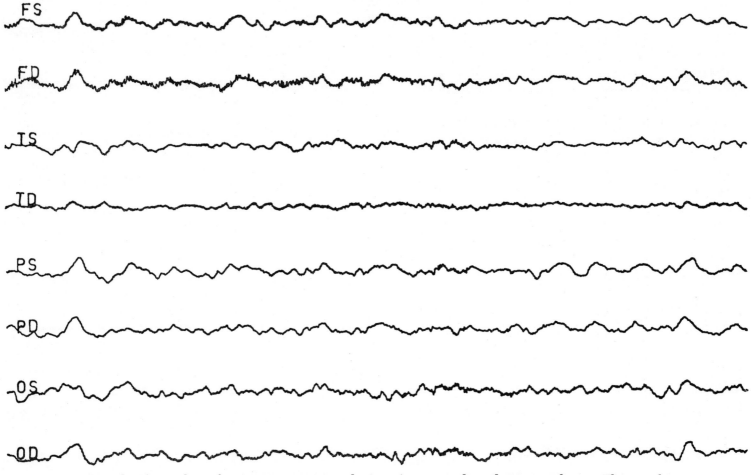

Irregular, low voltage frequencies, approximately 3 to 4 per second; moderate asynchrony. The asynchrony is normal in this period of life. Muscle artifacts in frontal leads.

FIGURE 2. — *One month, sleep.* 25

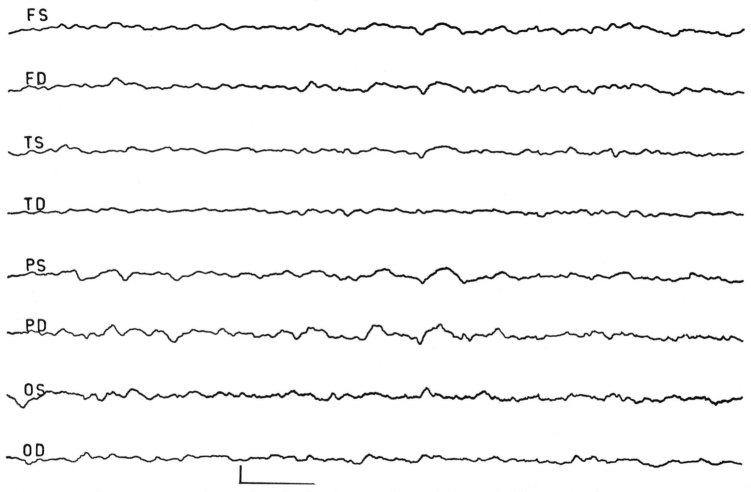

The same patient. The muscle artifact has disappeared. No fundamental difference between waking and sleep pattern. This is the type of tracing usually found at this age but occasionally spindles may be seen as early as the first month. The horizontal line indicates one second, the vertical line 50 microvolts.

FIGURE 3. — *Two months, awake.*

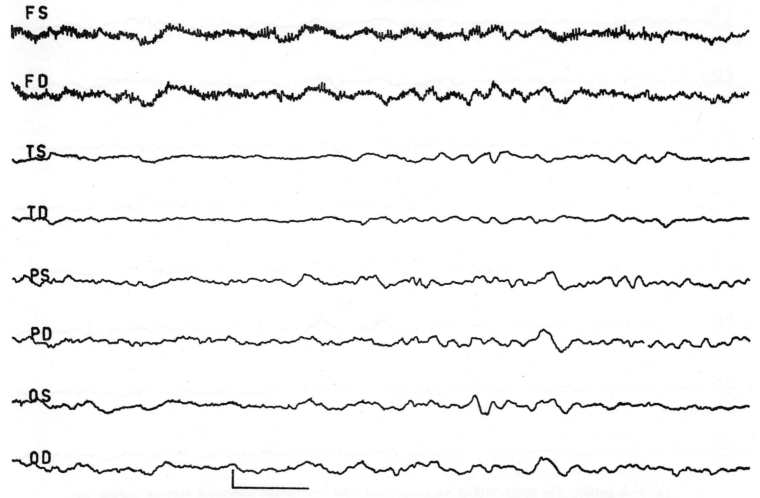

The frequency is similar to the one seen at one month but the voltage is higher. There still is asynchrony. Muscle artifact in frontal leads.

FIGURE 4. – *Two months, sleep.* 27

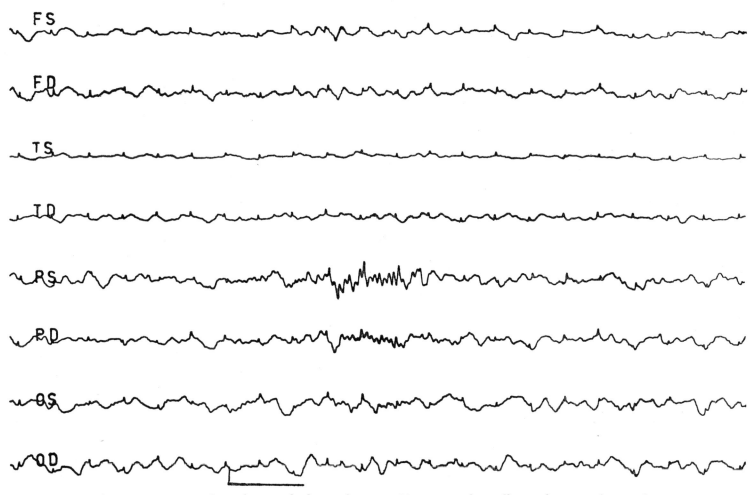

The same patient. The voltage is higher. There are 14 per second spindles in the parietal area; the asymmetry and asynchrony of the spindles is normal. The low voltage, sharp spikes are due to an incidentally recorded electrocardiogram; this is a common artifact in infants, especially when the diapers are wet.

FIGURE 5. — *Two months, arousal.*

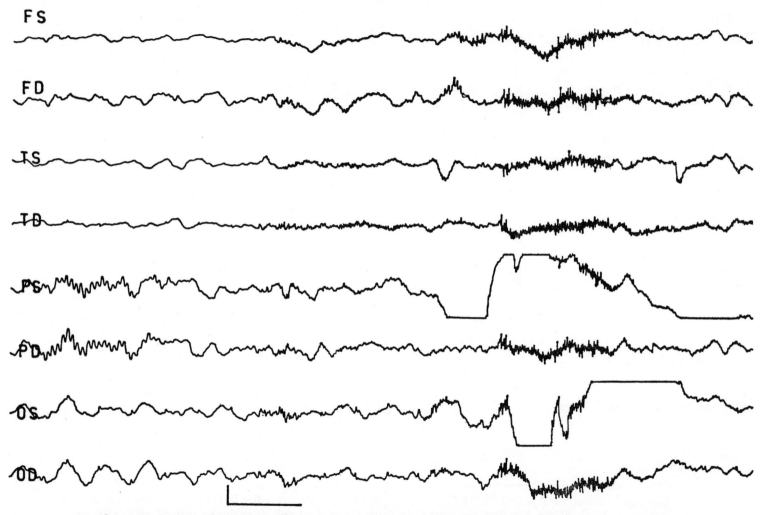

FS

FD

TS

TD

PS

PD

OS

OD

The same patient. The transition from sleep to waking is characterized by flattening of the waves and by the appearance of muscle artifacts.

FIGURE 6. — *Three months, awake.* 29

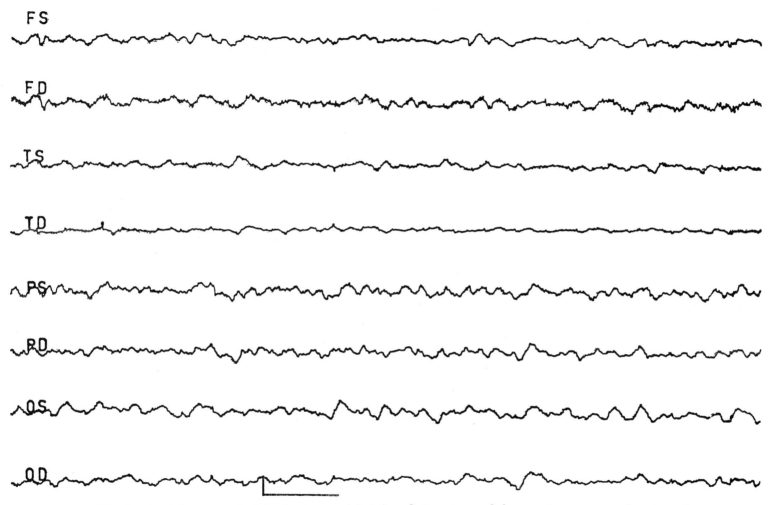

The dominant frequency is 3 to 4 per second but 5 and 6 per second frequencies are now also seen; the voltage is still rather low. Frontal muscle potentials.

FIGURE 7. — *Three months, sleep.*

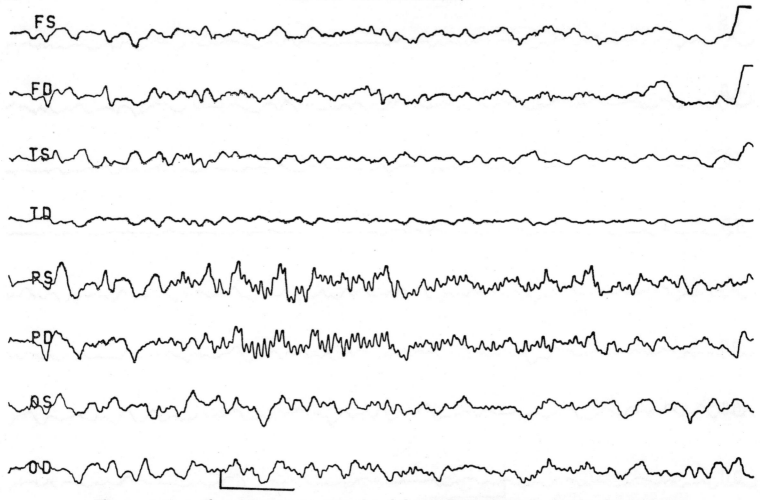

The same patient. The pattern is more organized, and the spindles are better developed and normally asynchronous.

FIGURE 8. — *Four months, awake.*   31

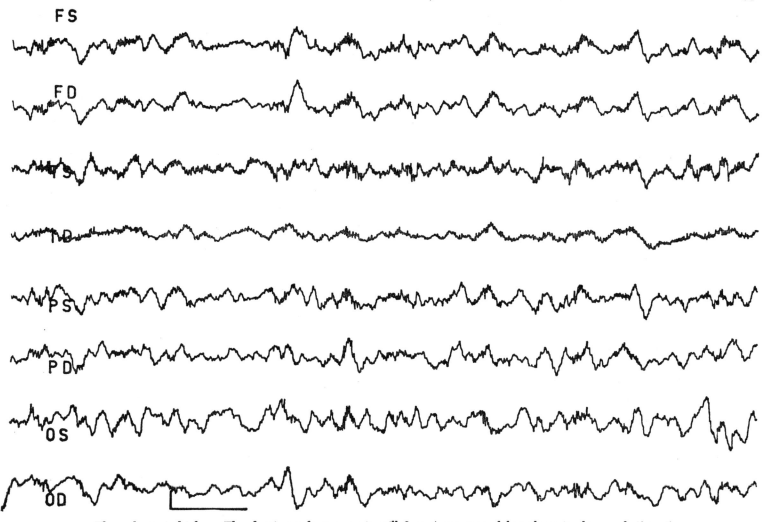

FIGURE 8. — *Four months, awake.*

The voltage is higher. The dominant frequency is still 3 to 4 per second but there is also much 5 to 7 per second activity, especially in the occipital leads. Both muscle potentials and some fast 25 to 30 per second activity are seen.

FIGURE 9. — *Four months, sleep.*

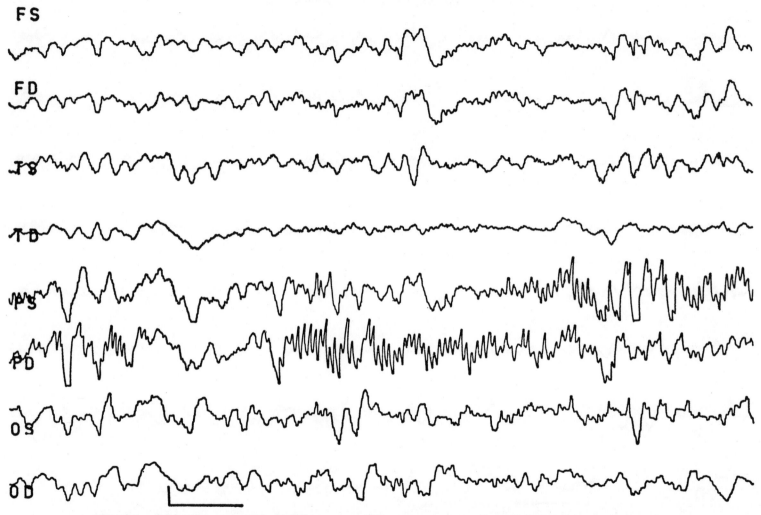

FS

FD

TS

TD

PS

PD

OS

OD

The same child. The tracings look different now. Fourteen per second parietal spindles are now well seen; the asynchrony is normal.

FIGURE 10. — *Four months, arousal.* 33

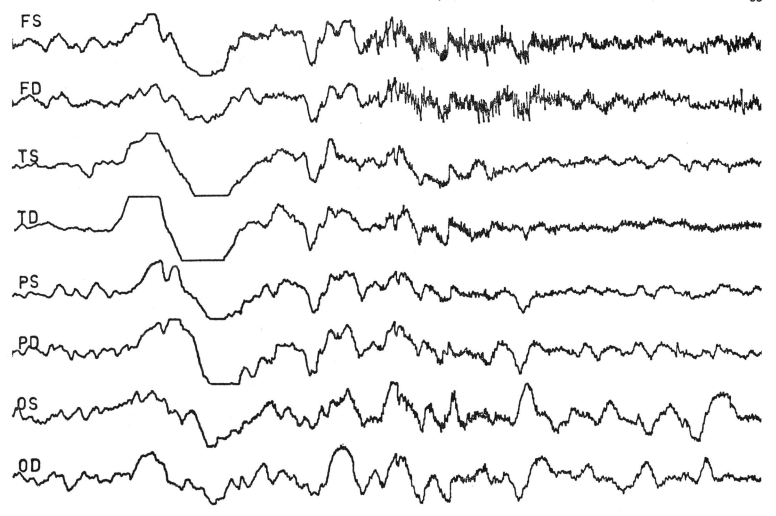

FS

FD

TS

TD

PS

PD

OS

OD

This phase is characterized by flattening of the tracing and by muscle movement artifacts.

FIGURE 11. — *Five months, awake.*

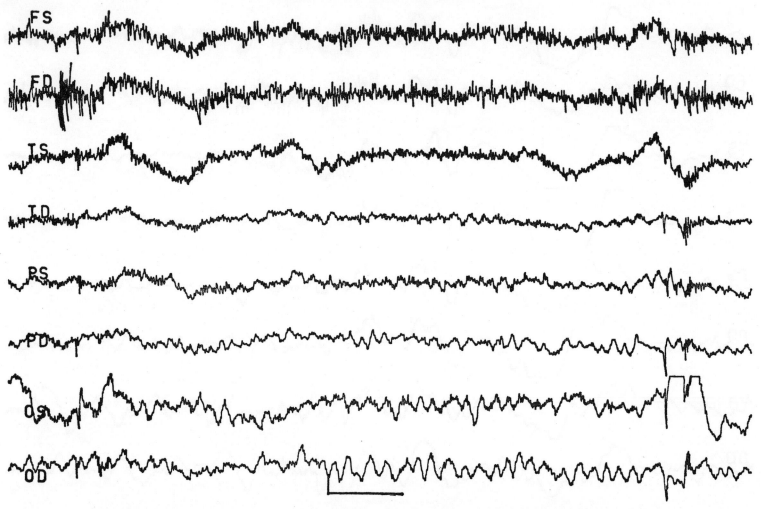

The basic frequency is 5 to 7 per second; muscle potentials are seen mostly in frontal and temporal areas.

Figure 12. — *Five months, sleep.*

35

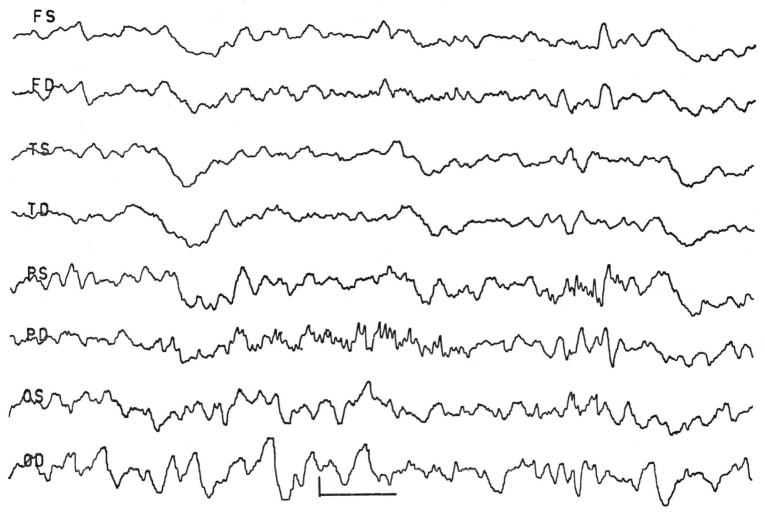

The same child. Regular slow 2 to 5 per second activity. Asynchrony is seen in the occipital leads and in the parietal spindles; it is normal in both areas.

FIGURE 13. — *Five months, arousal.*

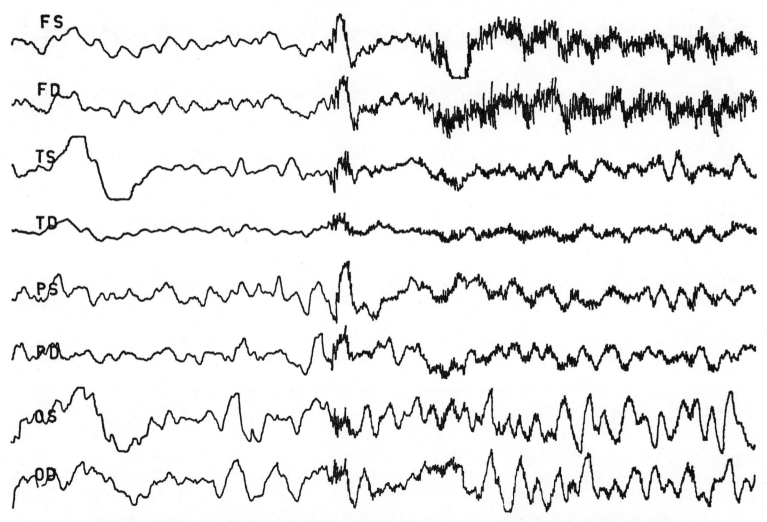

There is a tendency to the formation of slow paroxysmal features in the occipital leads. Superimposed muscle activity.

FIGURE 14. — *Six months, awake.* 37

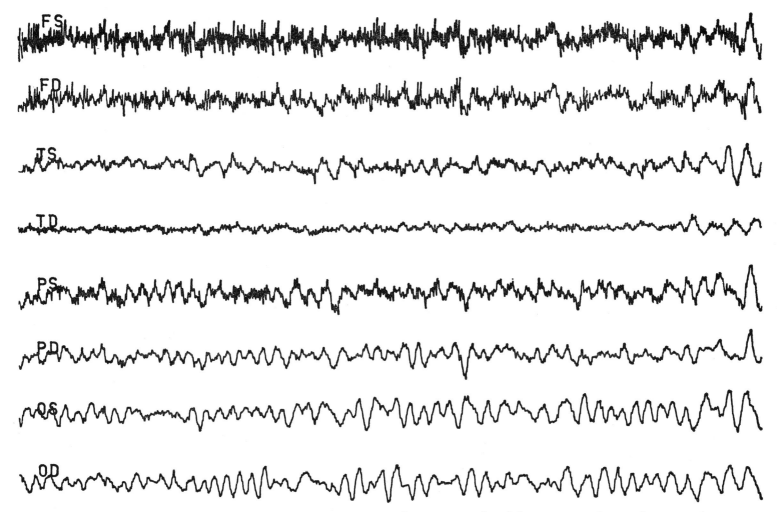

Five to 8 per second basic activity; the slowing on the extreme right of the picture is due to the onset of drowsiness. Muscle activity.

FIGURE 15. — *Six months, drowsy.*

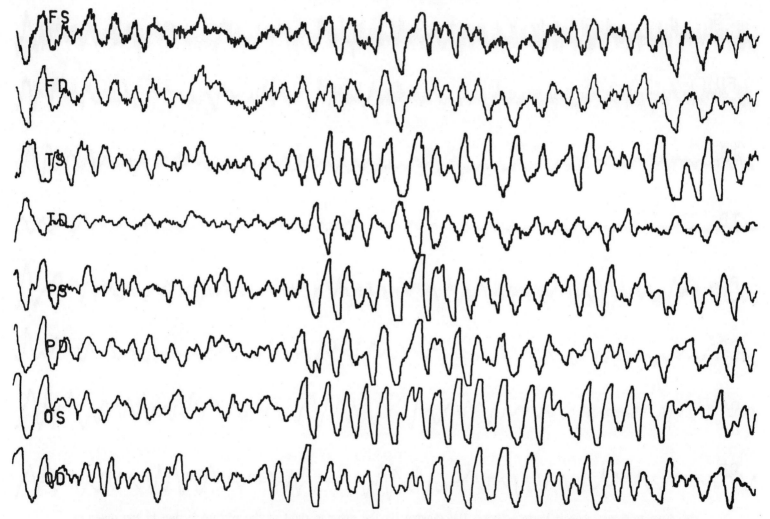

Appearance of 3 to 4 per second paroxysmal slowing; this is a normal phenomenon. Still some muscle activity of the forehead.

FIGURE 16. — *Six months, sleep.* 39

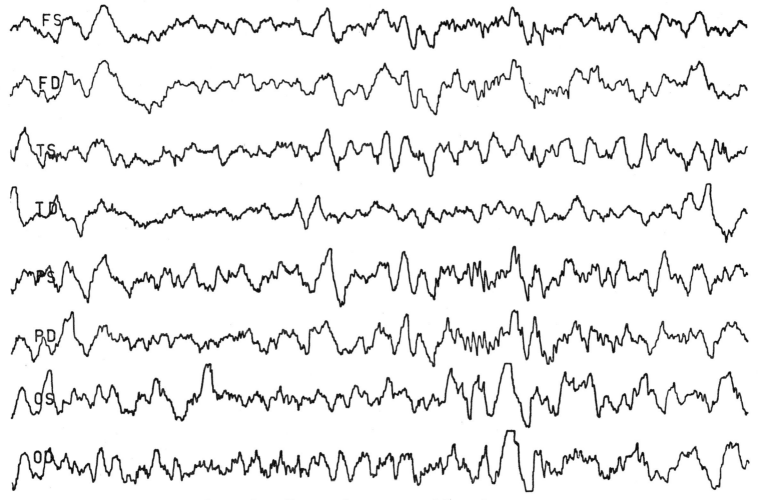

Fourteen per second parietal spindles; a moderate amount of low voltage 18 to 20 per second activity is superimposed on the usually asynchronous sleep pattern.

FIGURE 17. — *Six months, arousal.*

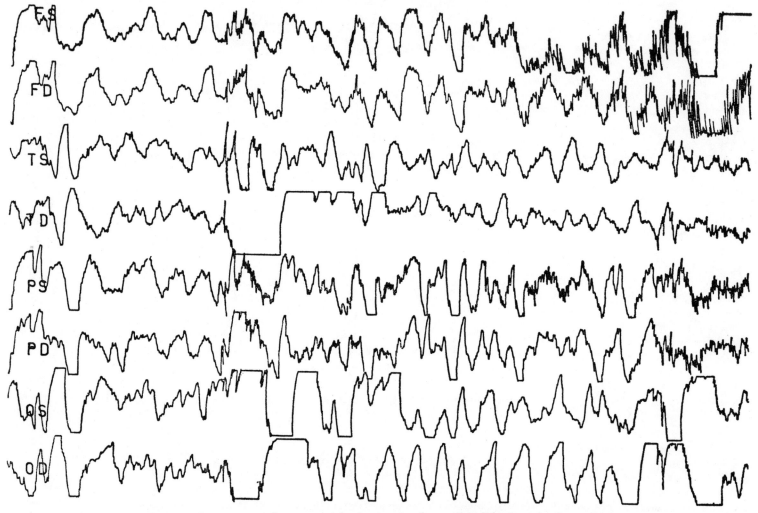

Two to 3 per second paroxysmal slowing in the occipital leads; muscle activity.

Figure 18. — *Seven months, awake.* 41

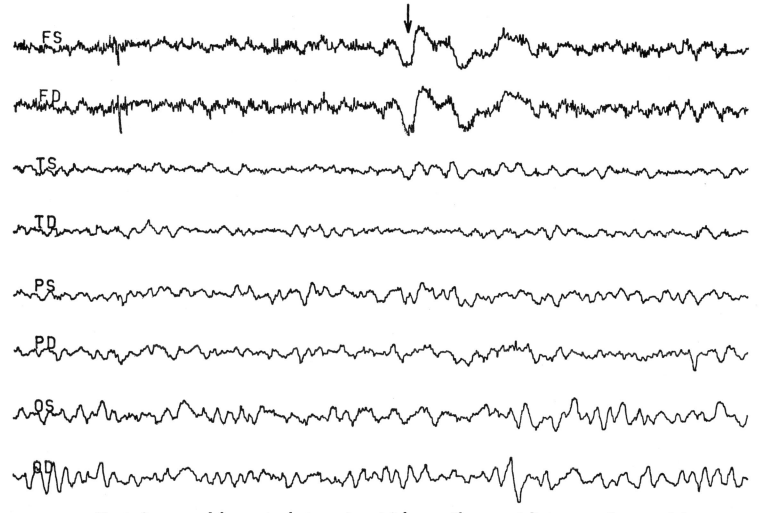

Five to 8 per second frequencies, best seen in occipital area. The arrow indicates an artifact caused by eye blinking.

FIGURE 19. — *Seven months, drowsy.*

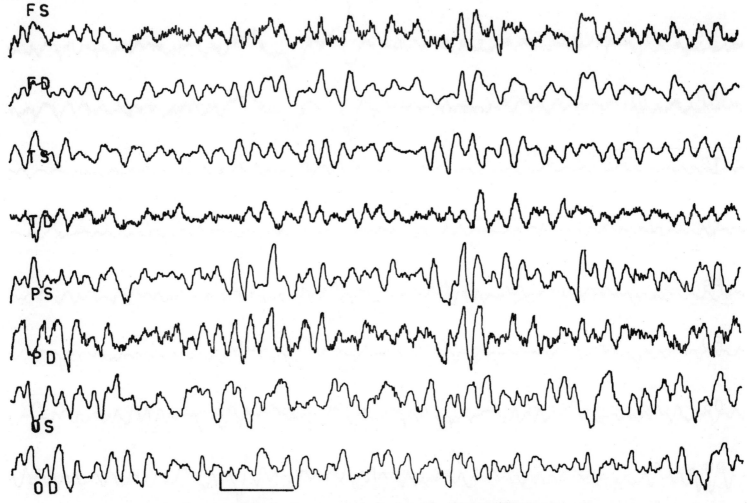

F S

F D

T S

T D

P S

P D

O S

O D

In the parietal leads, 3 per second slowing and rudimentary humps are seen.

FIGURE 20. — *Seven months, sleep.* 43

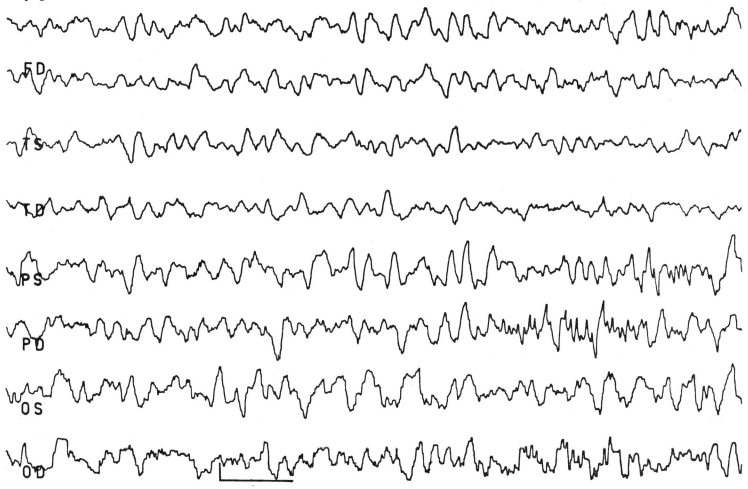

The same patient. Sleep frequencies are now very definite. Asynchronous 14 per second spindles in the parieto-occipital area.

44

FIGURE 21. — *Seven months, arousal.*

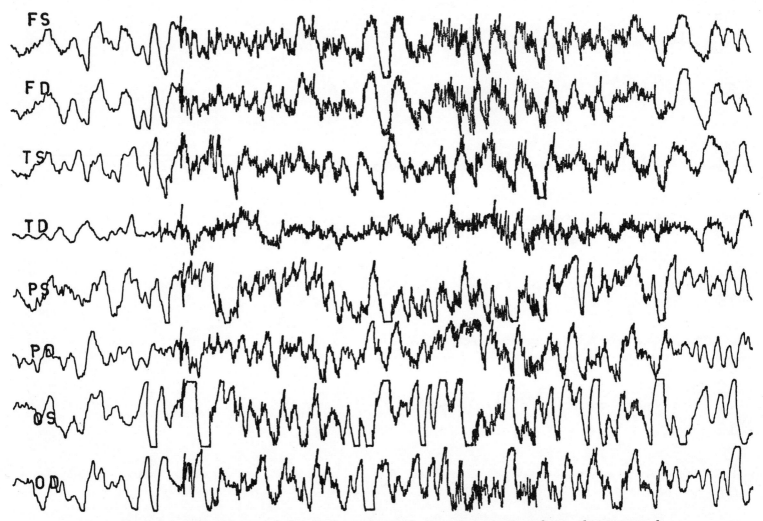

There is a diffuse slowing of the rhythm and asynchronous increase in voltage; this is normal.

FIGURE 22. — *Eight months, awake.* 45

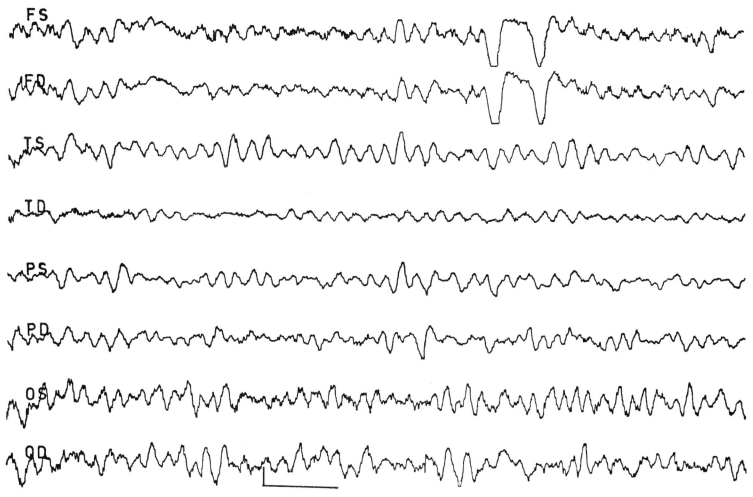

Five to 8 per second basic frequency, and 5 to 6 per second activity in temporal leads. The temporal asymmetry is normal with reference electrodes on the ears.

FIGURE 23. — *Eight months, drowsy.*

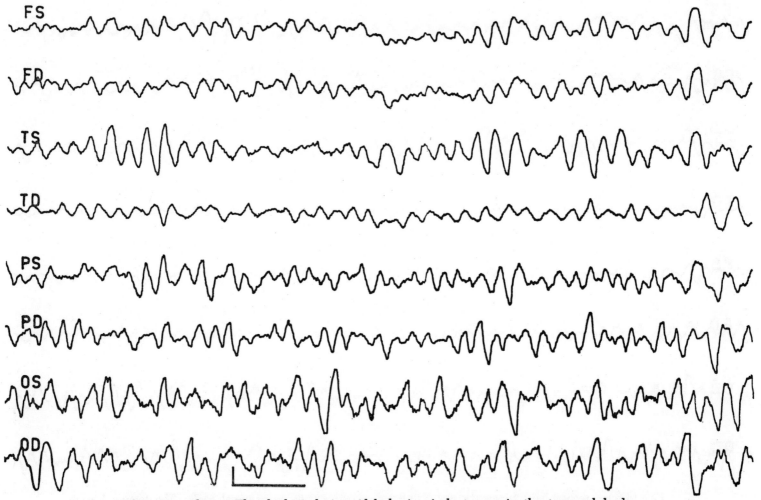

The same subject. The rhythmical sinusoidal slowing is best seen in the temporal leads.

FIGURE 24. — *Eight months, sleep.* 47

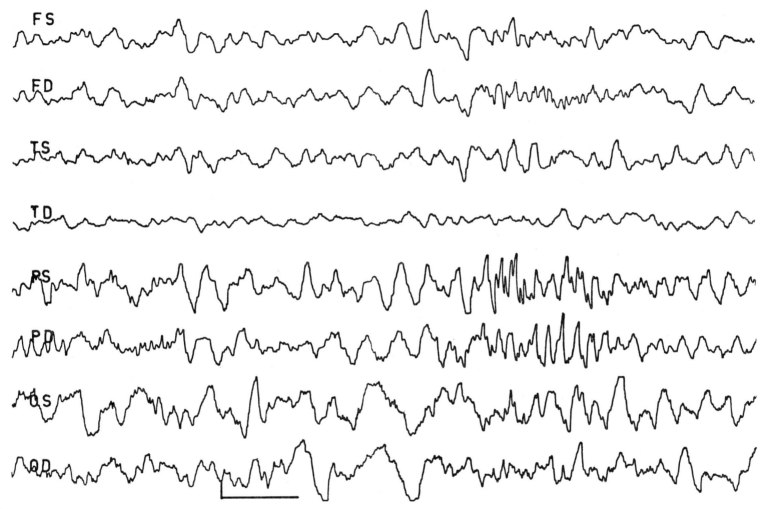

Spindle phase; the parietal spindles are higher, still asynchronous.

FIGURE 25. — *Eight months, arousal.*

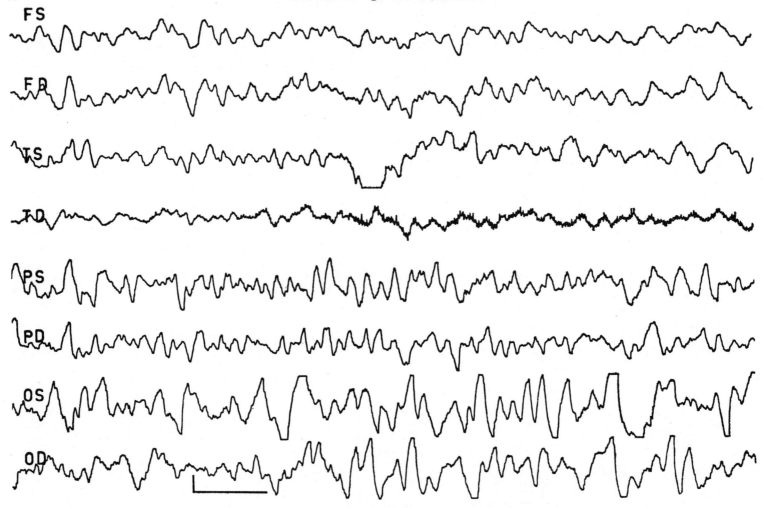

Tendency to synchronous slowing in occipital leads; muscle artifact appearing in right temporal lead.

FIGURE 26. — *Nine months, awake.* 49

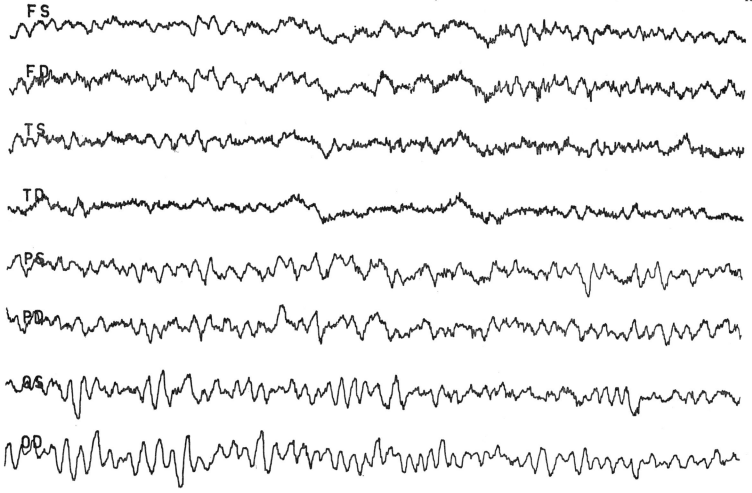

Six to 7 per second frequencies predominate but some 5 to 8 per second activity is also present. Superimposed muscle activity.

FIGURE 27. — *Nine months, drowsy.*

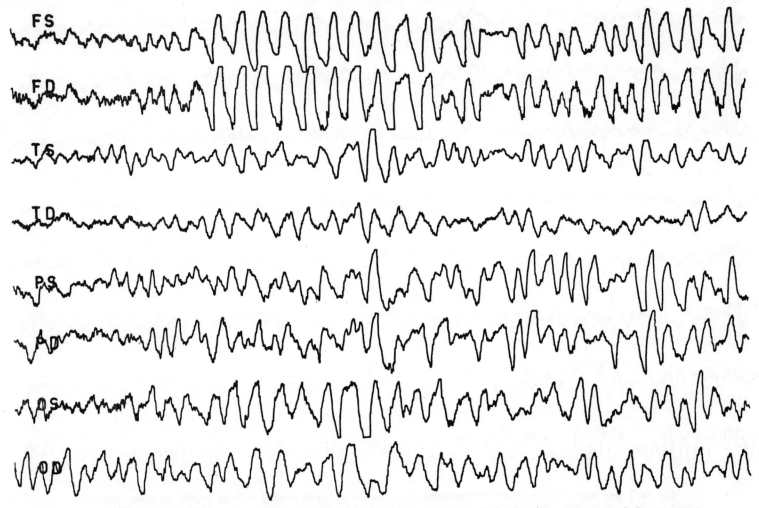

FS

FD

TS

TD

PS

AD

OS

OD

Three per second paroxysmal slow waves are best seen in the frontal leads. The interspersed fast activity can be mistaken for small spikes, but this is normal in this age group.

FIGURE 28. — *Nine months, sleep.* 51

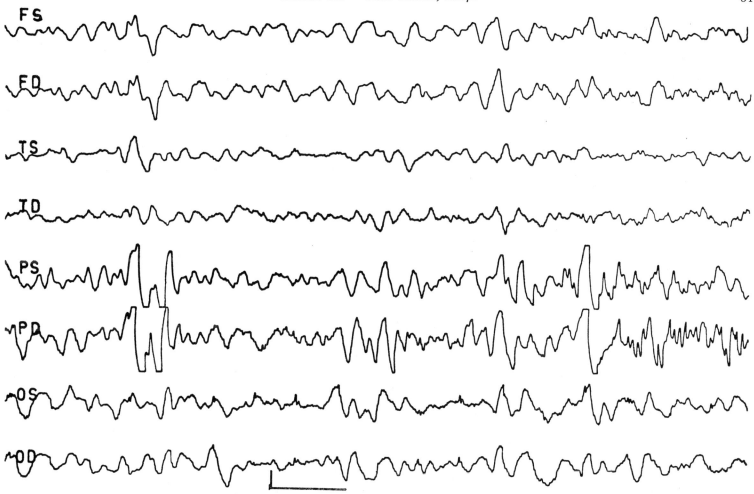

In the parietal leads, well formed humps are seen; they precede the spindles.

FIGURE 29. — *Nine months, arousal.*

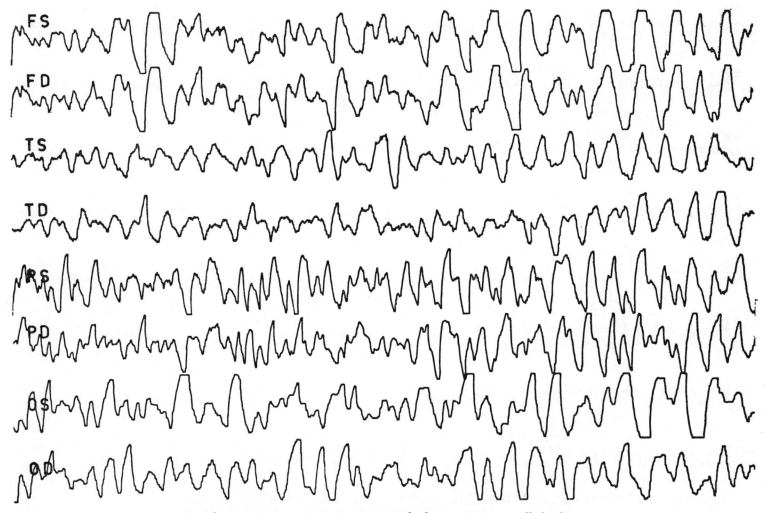

Regular, continuous 2 to 4 per second slow activity in all leads.

Figure 30. — *Ten and one-half months, awake.*
53

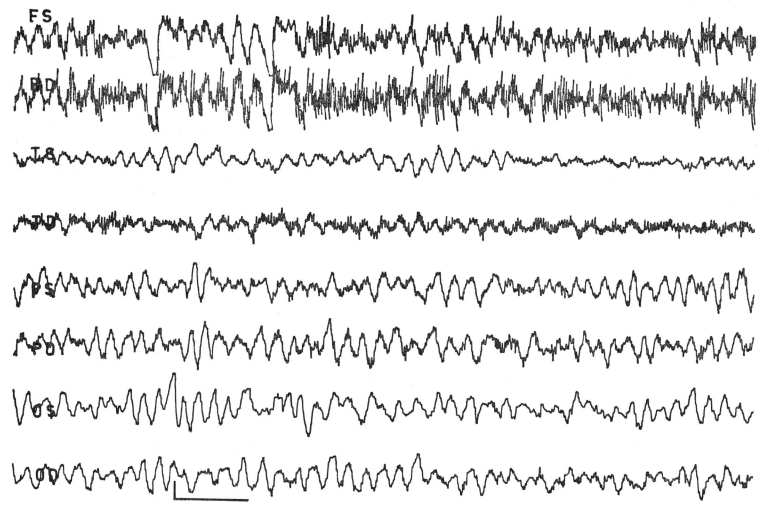

Five to 8 per second basic activity. Blinking and muscle artifacts in frontal leads.

FIGURE 31. — *Ten months, drowsy.*

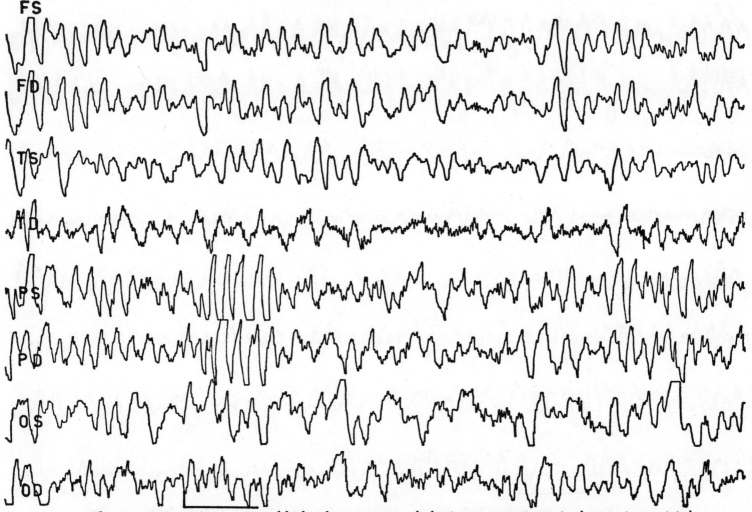

The same patient. Appearances of high voltage, paroxysmal slowing may at times simulate parieto-occipital spikes; superimposed 20 to 25 per second activity. It should be emphasized that above paroxysmal pattern is normal at this age.

FIGURE 32. — *Ten months, arousal.* 55

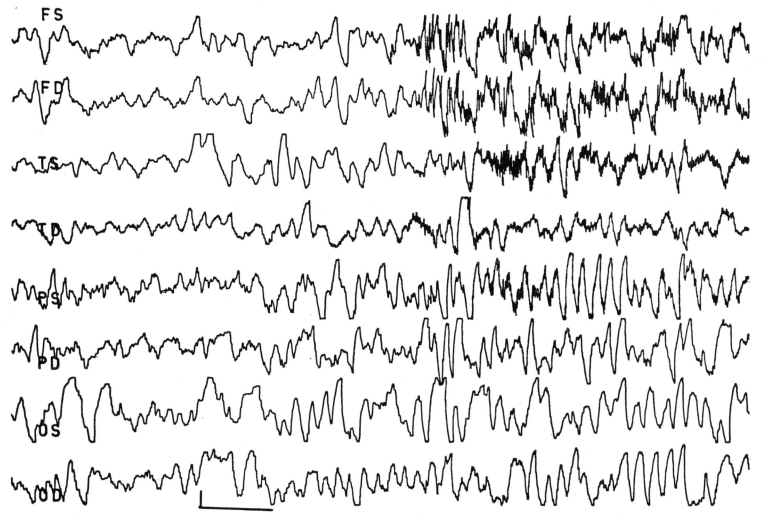

High voltage, 3 to 5 per second paroxysmal slowing in all leads.

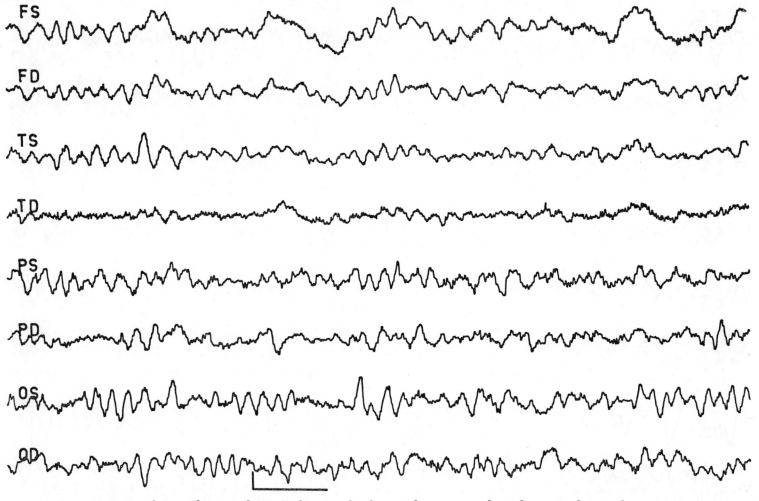

FIGURE 33. — *Ten and one-half months, awake.*

Transition from waking to sleep. Reduction of voltage is best seen in the right occipital-parietal area. Some low voltage 15 to 18 per second fast activity.

FIGURE 34. — *Ten and one-half months, drowsy.* 57

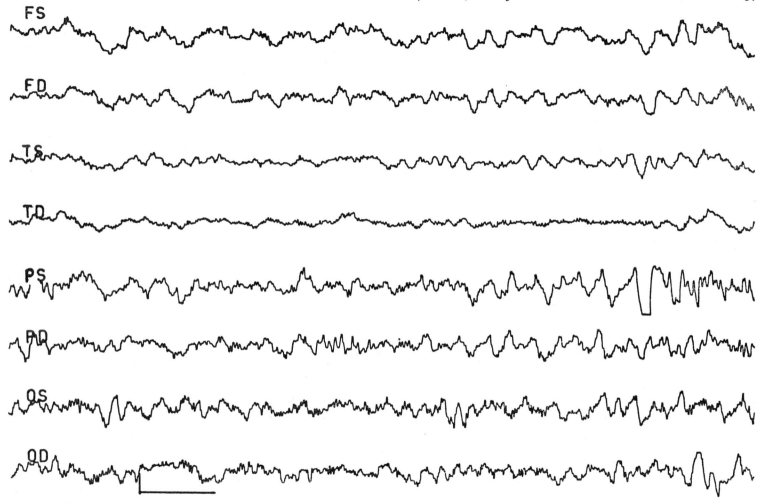

Further reduction of voltage with 20 to 22 per second occipital frequencies. Spindles are appearing in the parietal leads. This fast activity during drowsiness is normal at this age.

FIGURE 35. — *Eleven months, awake.*

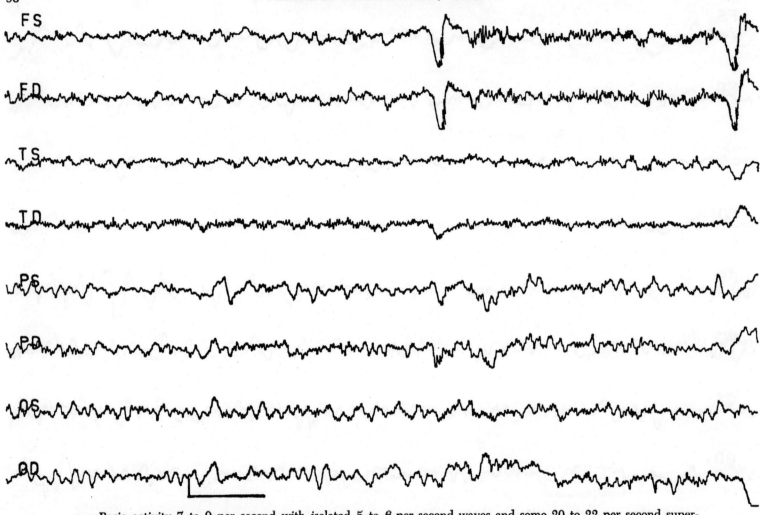

Basic activity 7 to 9 per second with isolated 5 to 6 per second waves and some 20 to 22 per second superimposed frequencies. Blinking artifacts in frontal leads.

FIGURE 36. — *Eleven months, sleep.* 59

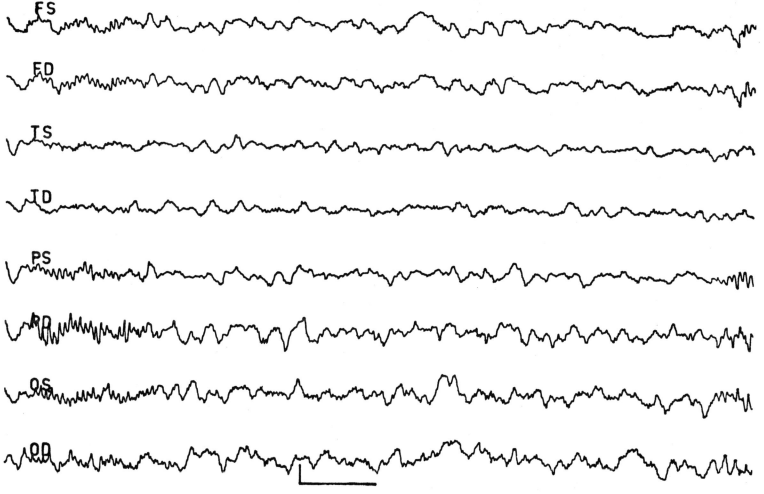

The same child. Synchronous 14 per second spindles in all leads.

FIGURE 37. — *Eleven months, deep sleep.*

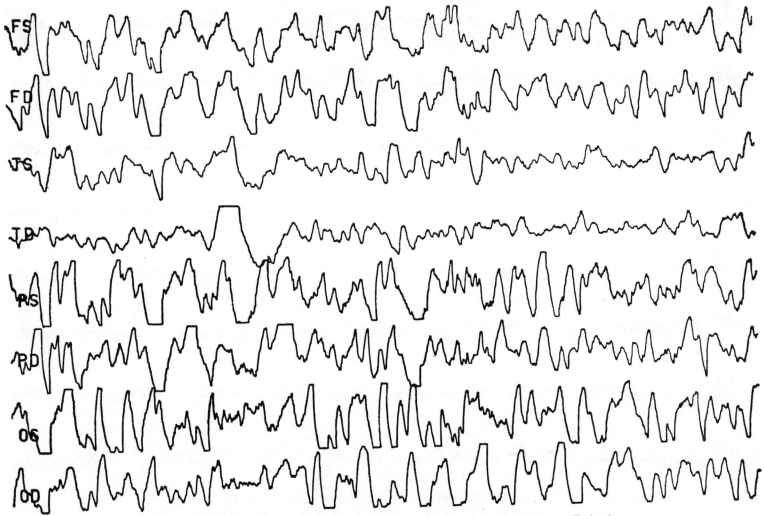

The same child. Slow, irregular, polymorphous high voltage waves in all leads.

FIGURE 38. — *Eleven months, arousal.* 61

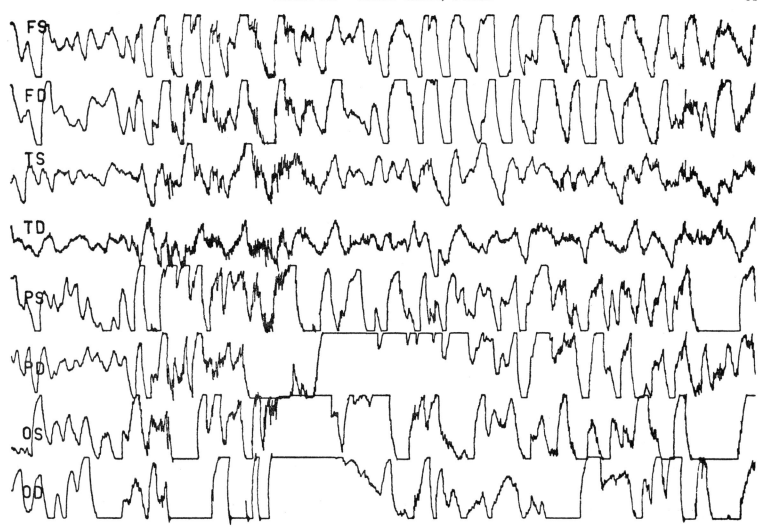

The same child. Appearance of slow, regular, paroxysmal, rhythms. This slowing may last tens of seconds.

FIGURE 39. — *Twelve months, awake.*

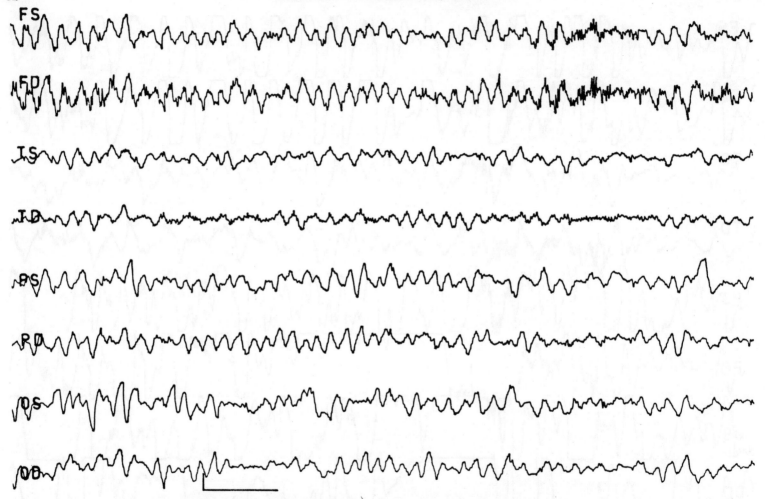

Basic 5 to 8 per second activity in all leads with some frontal 20 to 25 per second waves in the frontal area.

FIGURE 40. — *Twelve months, asleep.* 63

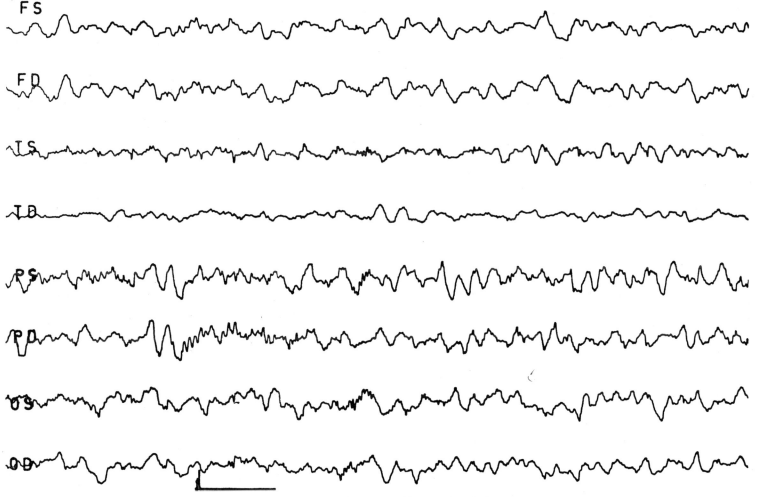

FS

FD

IS

ID

PS

PD

OS

OD

The same patient. Low voltage spindles with slight asynchrony.

FIGURE 41. — *Twelve months, arousal.*

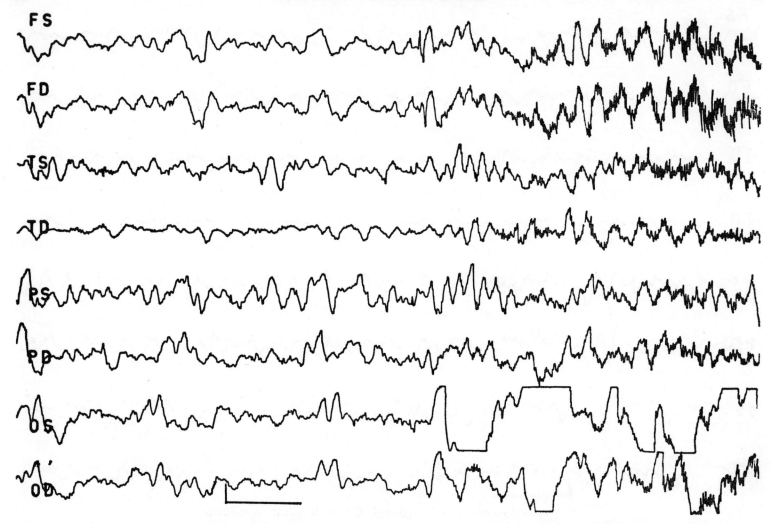

FS

FD

TS

TD

PS

PD

OS

OD

Five to 6 per second paroxysmal activity of slow duration; muscle artifacts.

FIGURE 42. — *Twenty-one months, awake.* 65

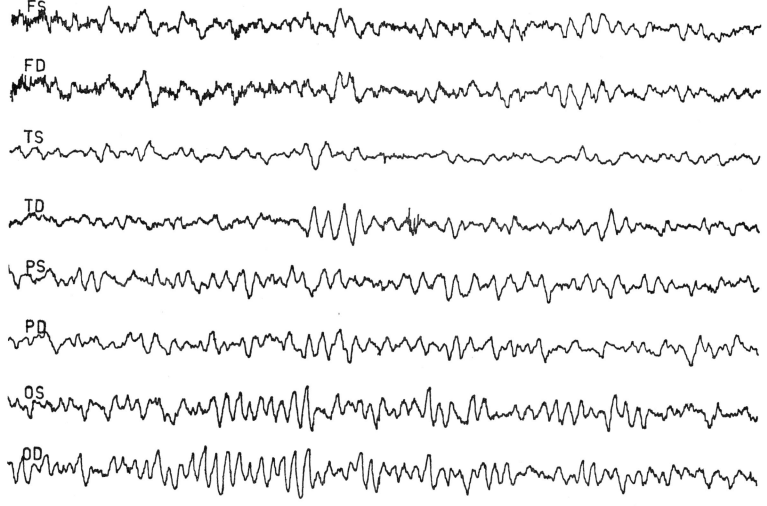

Basic activity 6 to 8 per second, best seen in occipital leads.

FIGURE 43. — *Fourteen months, drowsy.*

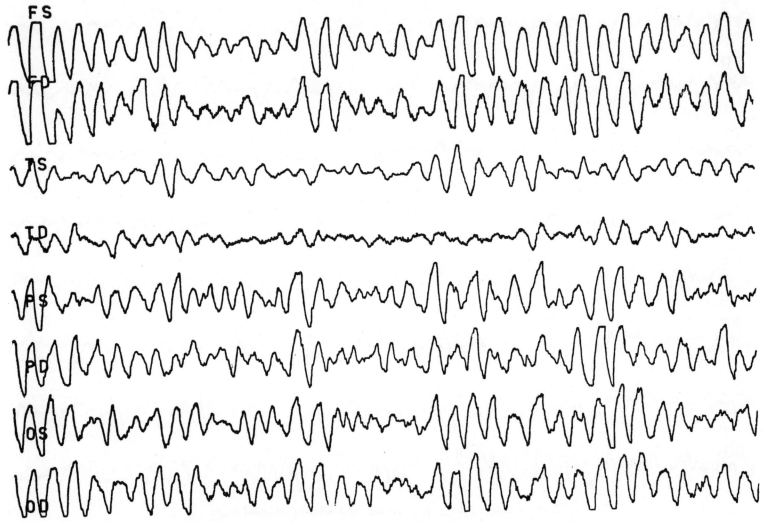

Paroxysmal, 3 per second slow wave activity; this is perfectly normal.

FIGURE 44. — *Sixteen months, very light sleep.* 67

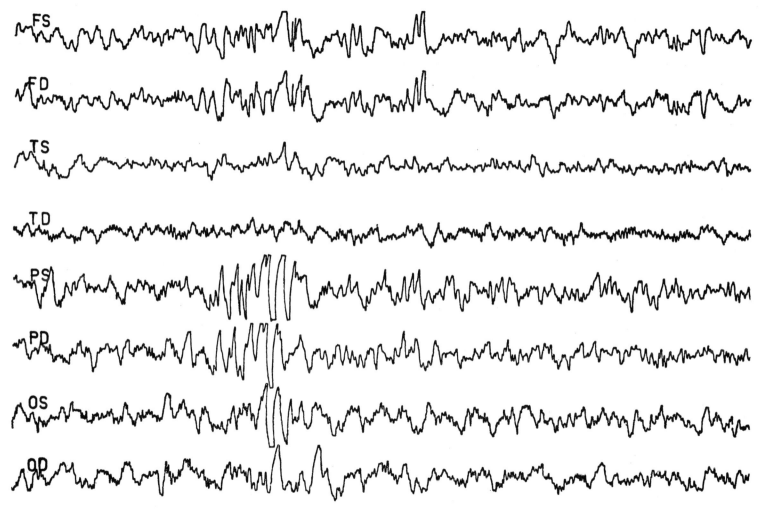

Synchronous, high voltage humps in parietal leads and a moderate amount of diffuse 20 to 25 per second fast activity.

FIGURE 45. — *Sixteen months, sleep.*

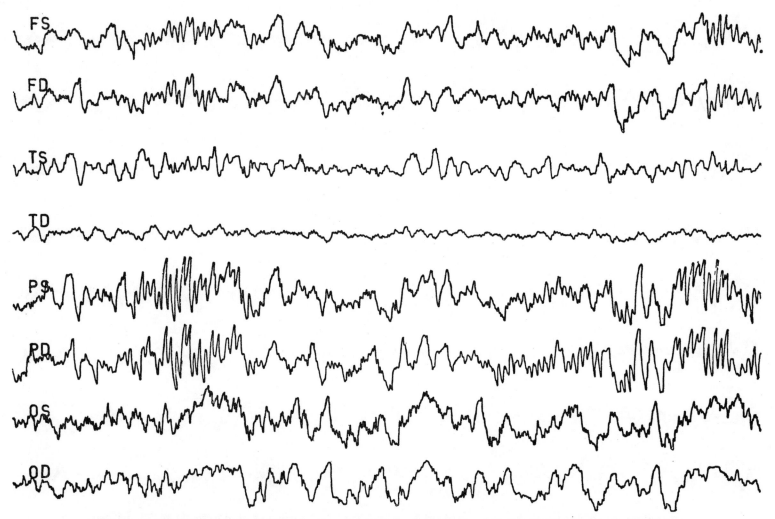

The same patient. Twelve to 14 per second spindles in parietal and frontal leads; fast activity is less common in this stage of sleep.

FIGURE 46. — *Sixteen months, arousal.* 69

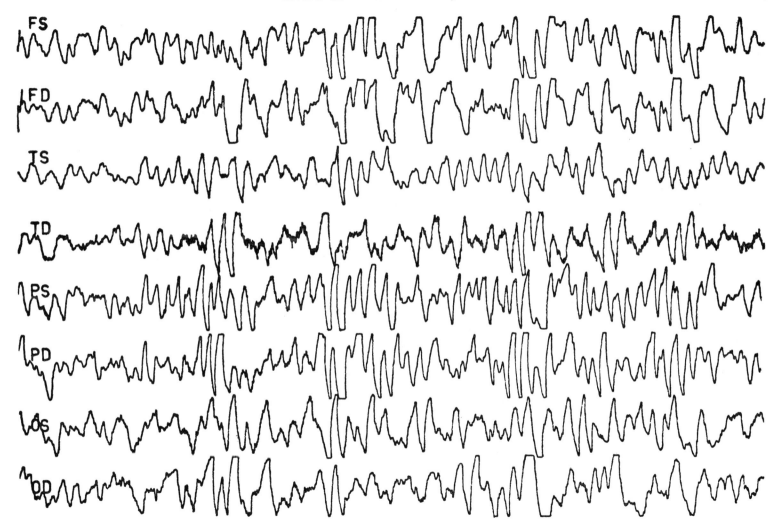

The same patient. Paroxysmal, high voltage 3 to 6 per second activity.

FIGURE 47. — *Two years, awake.*

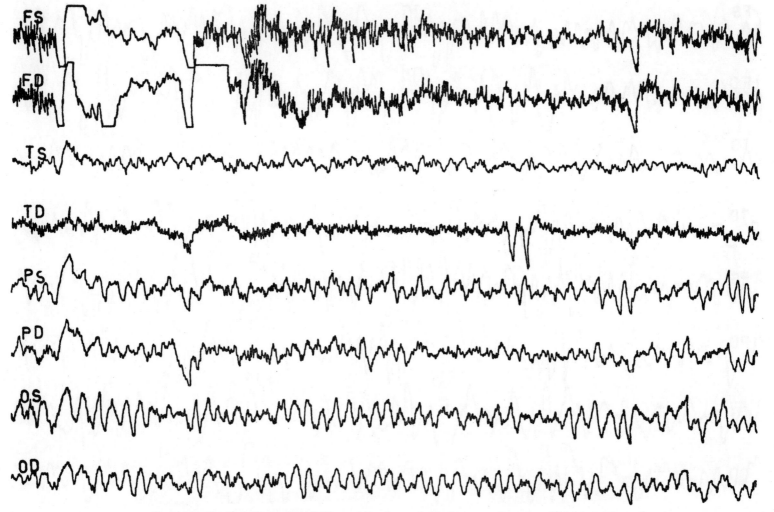

Six to 8 per second regular rhythm. Muscle and blinking artifacts in frontal leads.

FIGURE 48. — *Two years, drowsy.* 71

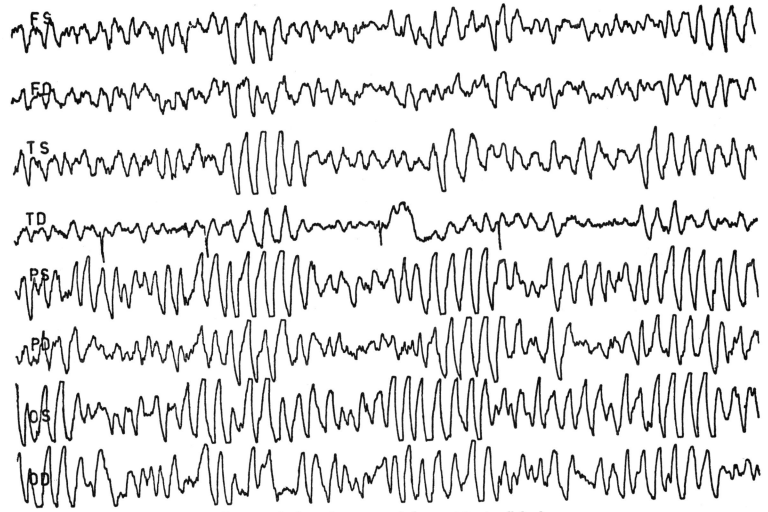

Paroxysmal, 3 to 4 per second slow activity in all leads.

FIGURE 49. — *Two years, sleep.*

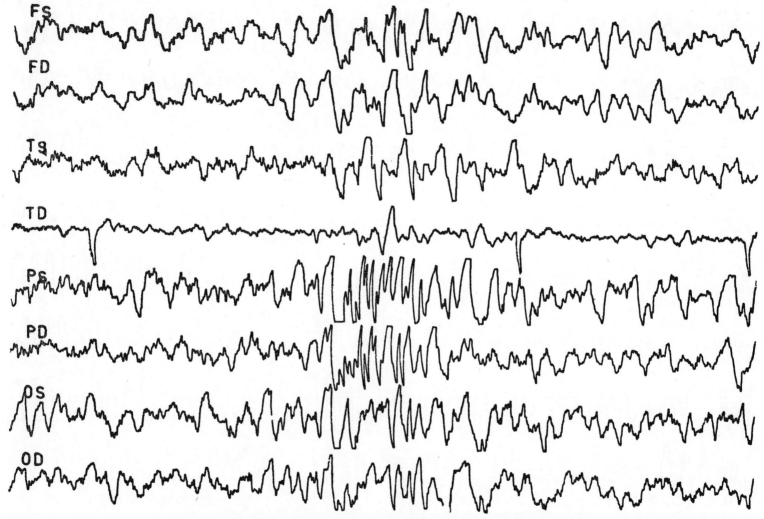

FS

FD

TS

TD

PS

PD

OS

OD

The same patient. High voltage humps and synchronous sharp spindles.

FIGURE 50. — *Two years, arousal.* 73

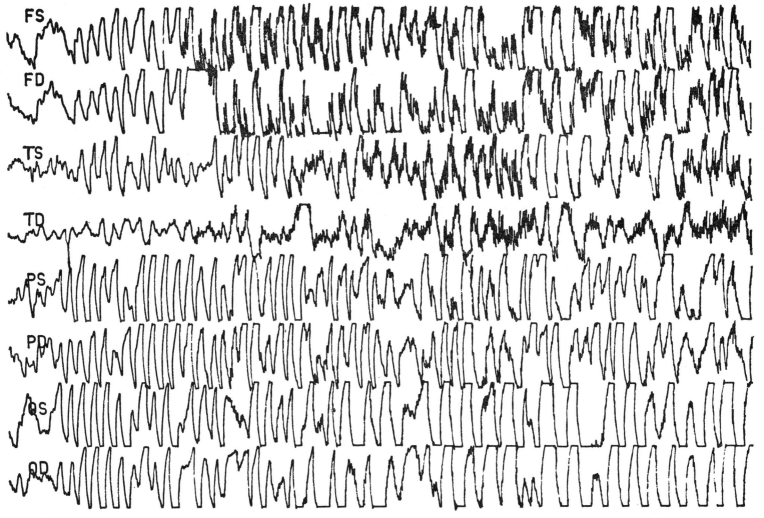

The same patient. Continuous, paroxysmal 3 to 4 per second activity.

FIGURE 51. — *Three years, awake.*

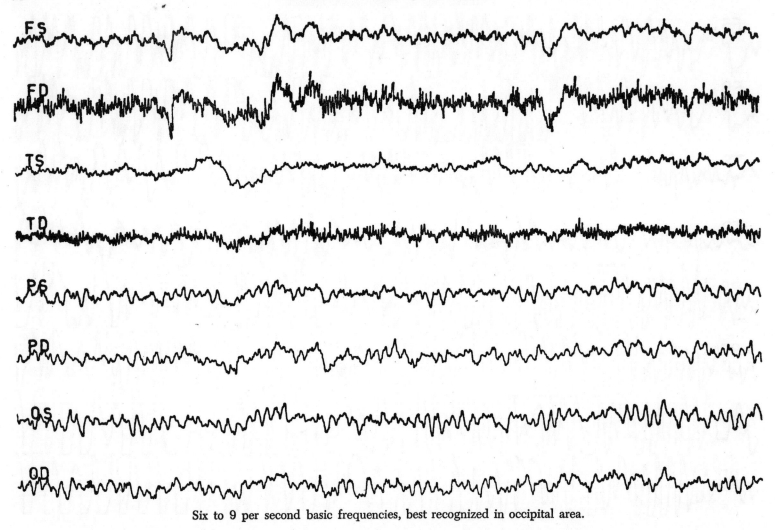

Six to 9 per second basic frequencies, best recognized in occipital area.

FIGURE 52. — *Three years, arousal.* 75

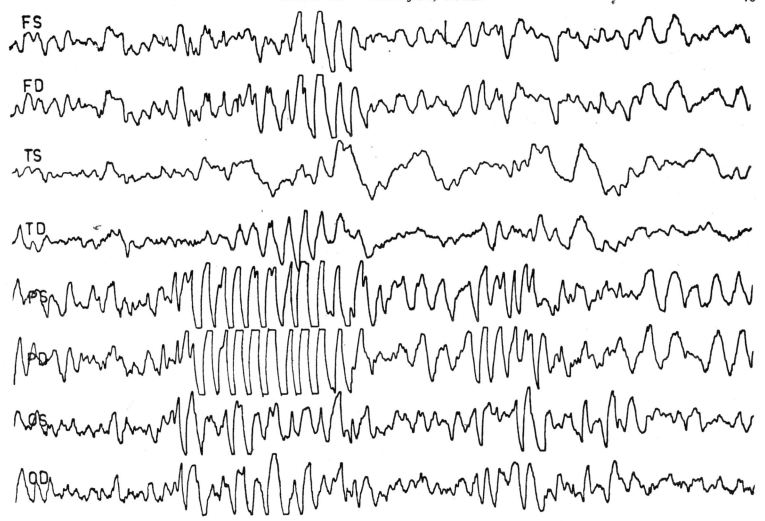

The same patient. The paroxysmal slow activity of drowsiness is of shorter duration at this age and is interspersed by very low voltage waves.

FIGURE 53. — *Three years, sleep.*

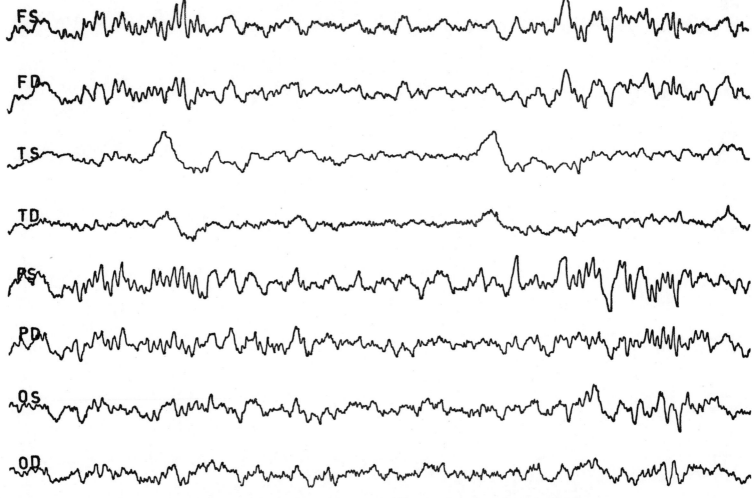

Twelve to 14 per second synchronous spindles in frontal and parietal lobes.

FIGURE 54. — *Three years, arousal.*

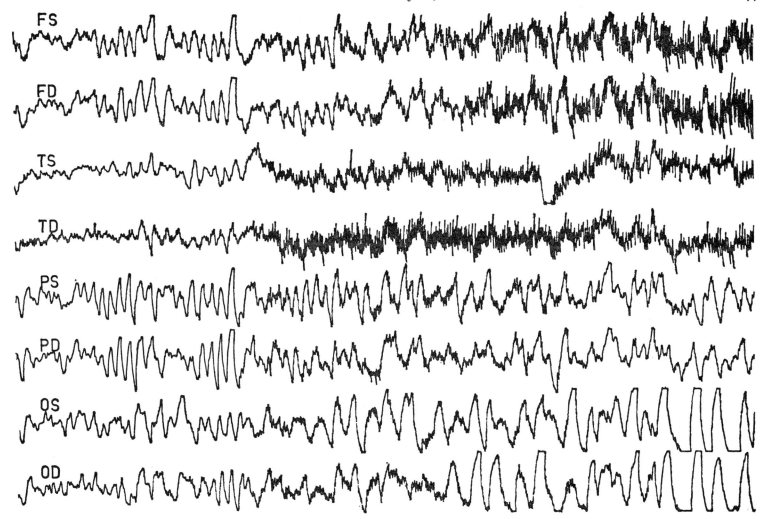

FS
FD
TS
TD
PS
PD
OS
OD

Paroxysmal 7 to 8 per second, high voltage activity with runs of 3 to 4 per second waves in the occipital leads. Muscle potentials in frontal and temporal areas.

FIGURE 55. — *Four and one-half years, awake.*

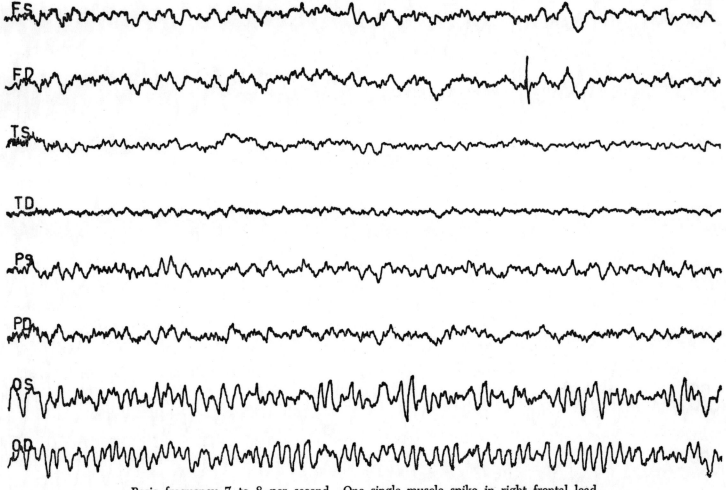

Basic frequency 7 to 8 per second. One single muscle spike in right frontal lead.

FIGURE 56. — *Four and one-half years, light sleep.* 79

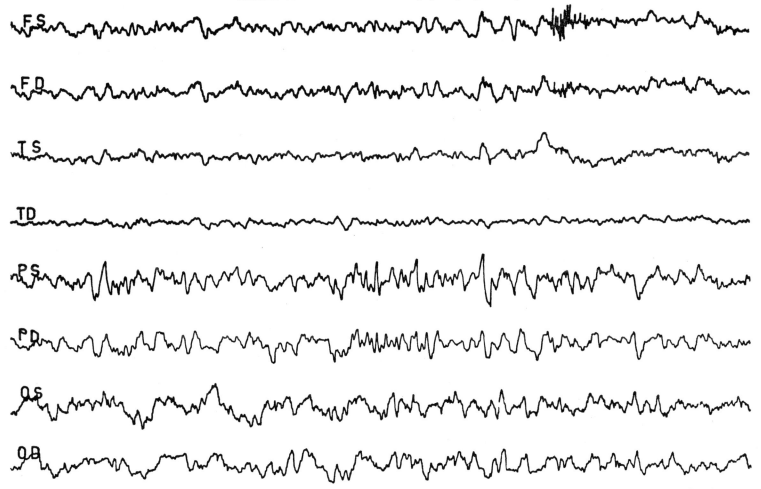

The same patient. Humps and low voltage 14 per second spindles in the parietal leads; still some muscle artifact from forehead.

FIGURE 57. — *Four and one-half years, sleep.*

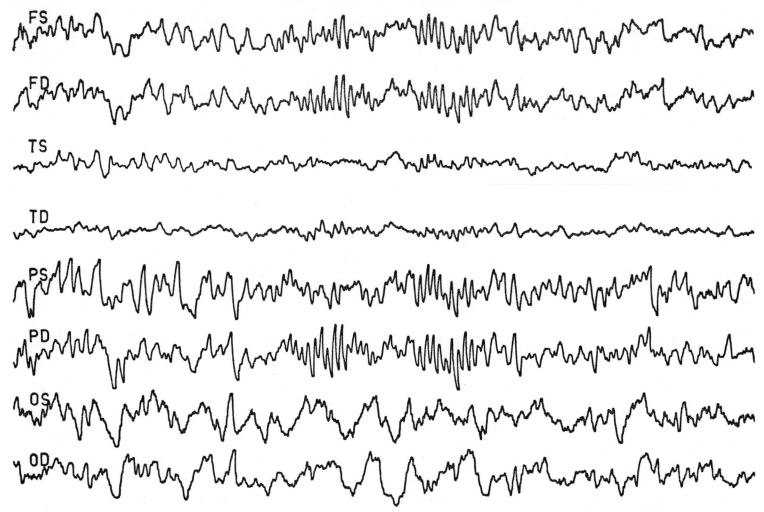

The same patient. The humps are clearly seen, and the spindles are of higher voltage in this stage of sleep.

FIGURE 58. — *Four and one-half years, arousal.* 81

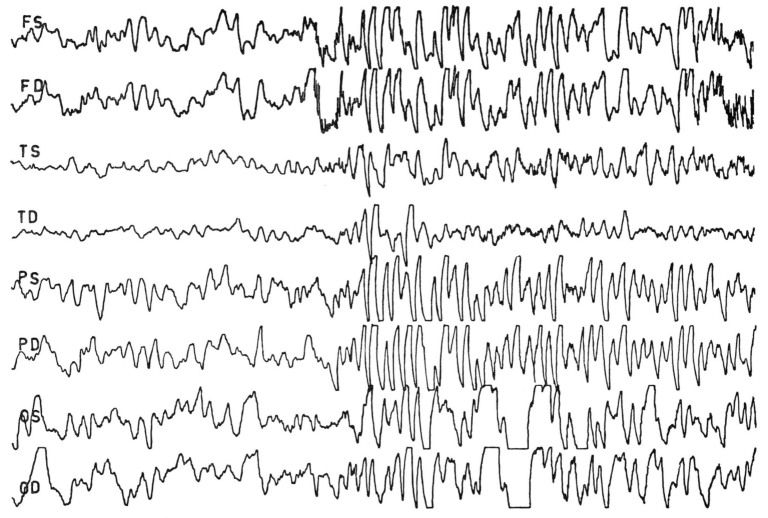

Paroxysmal 6 to 7 per second waves with some 3 to 4 per second activity in occipital leads.

FIGURE 59. — *Five years, awake.*

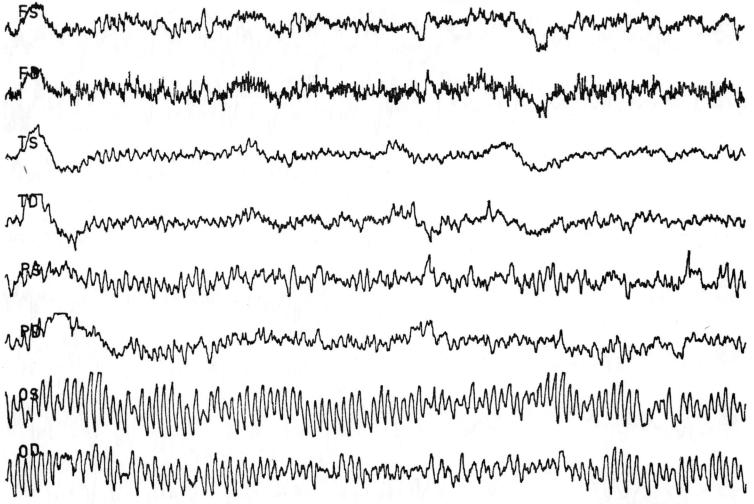

Well developed, 9 to 10 per second basic activity in occipital leads; the waves are very sharp in the parietal leads.

Figure 60. — *Five years, light sleep.* 83

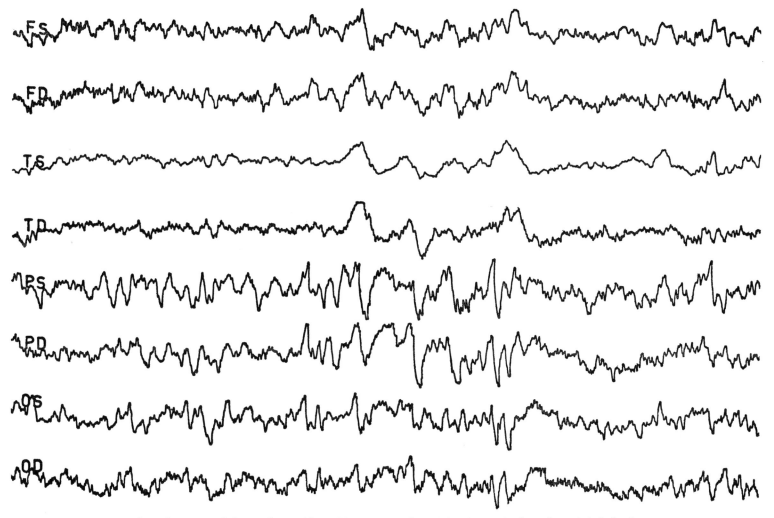

Sleep humps and low voltage 18 to 22 per second activity in parietal and occipital leads.

FIGURE 61. — *Five years, deep sleep.*

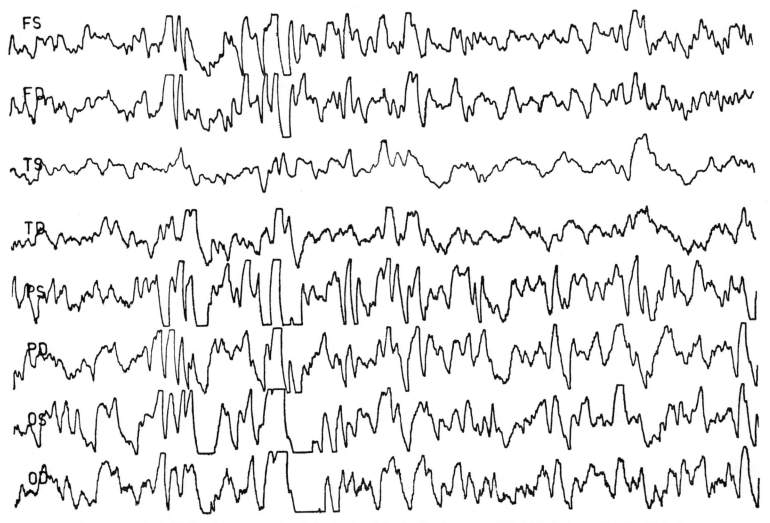

FS

FD

TS

TD

PS

PD

OS

OD

The same patient. High voltage, paroxysmal slowing in all leads; the sharp waves should not be confused with spikes.

FIGURE 62. — *Five years, arousal.* 85

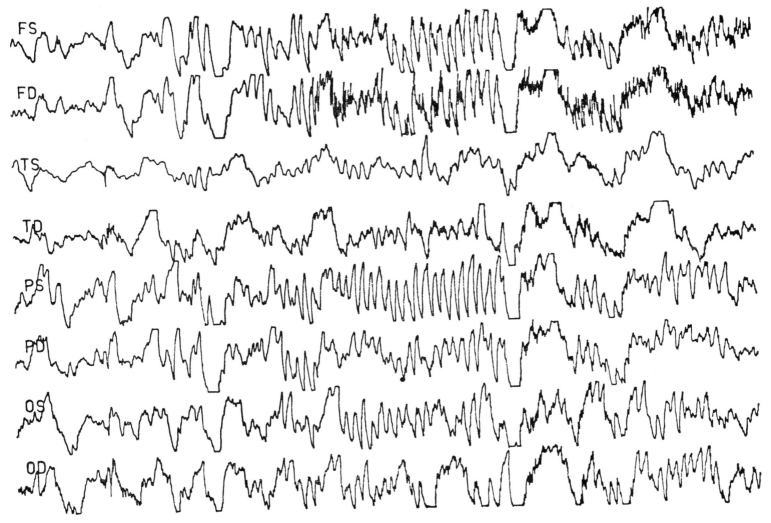

Paroxysms of 6 to 7 per second waves of short duration constitute a normal arousal pattern.

FIGURE 63. — *Six years, awake.*

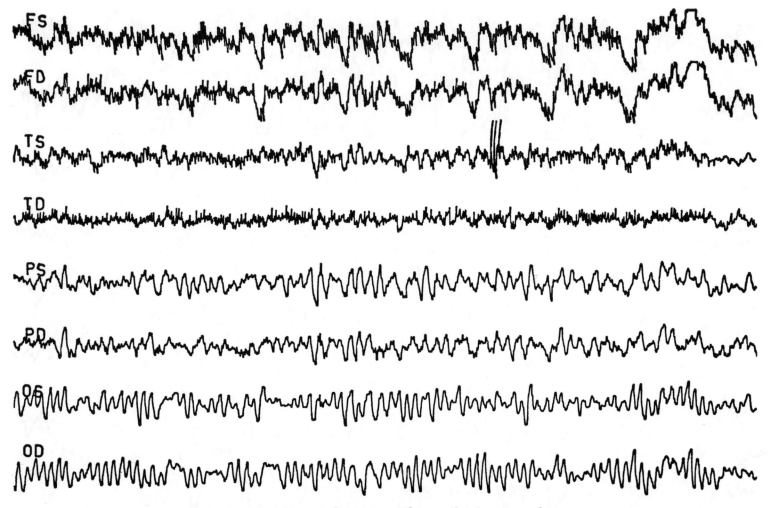

Basic 8 to 9 per second activity with some 5 to 6 per second waves.

FIGURE 64. — *Six years, drowsy.* 87

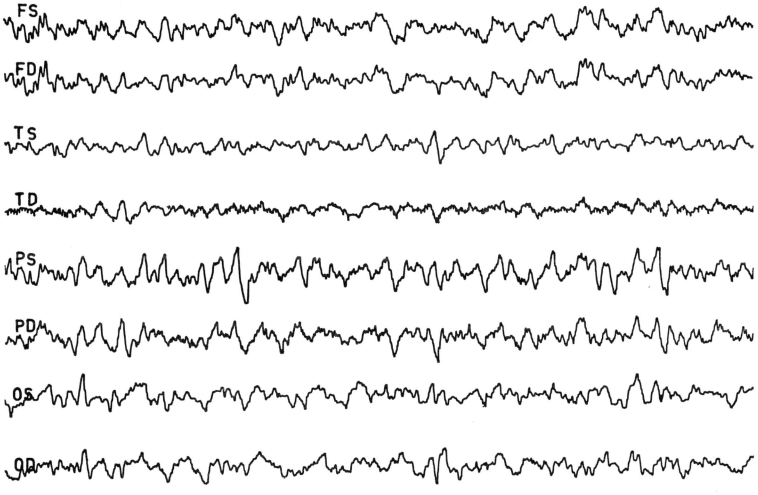

Lower voltage; a few, isolated, parietal humps.

FIGURE 65. — *Six years, sleep.*

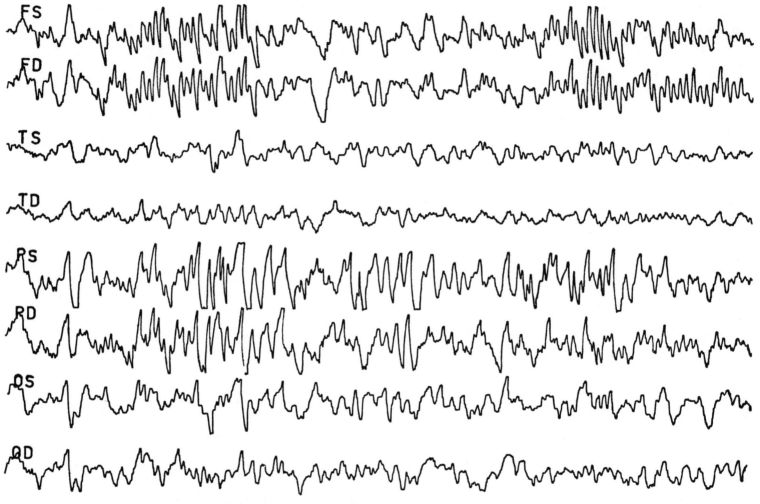

FS

FD

TS

TD

RS

RD

OS

OD

Many high voltage, synchronous humps and fragmentary 14 per second spindles in parietal leads; sharp spindles of approximately 12 per second frequency in frontal area.

FIGURE 66. — *Six year, arousal.* 89

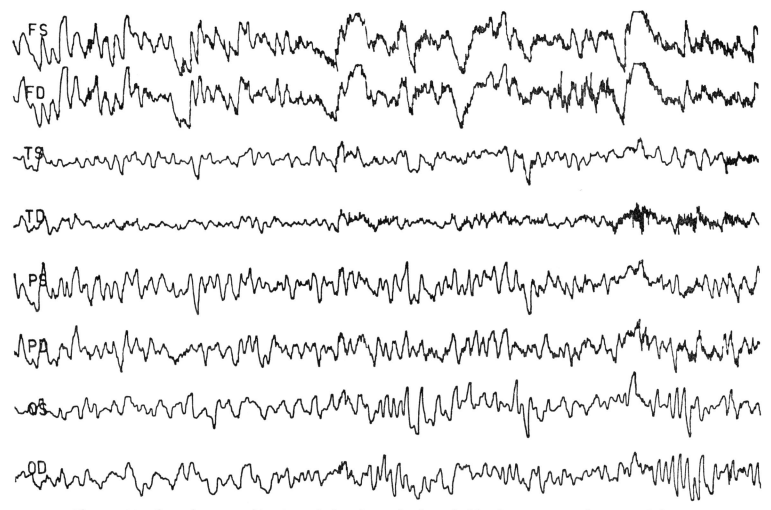

FS

FD

TS

TD

PS

PD

OS

OD

The transition from sleep to waking is gradual and not clearly marked by the appearance of paroxysmal slowing.

FIGURE 67. — *Seven years, awake.*

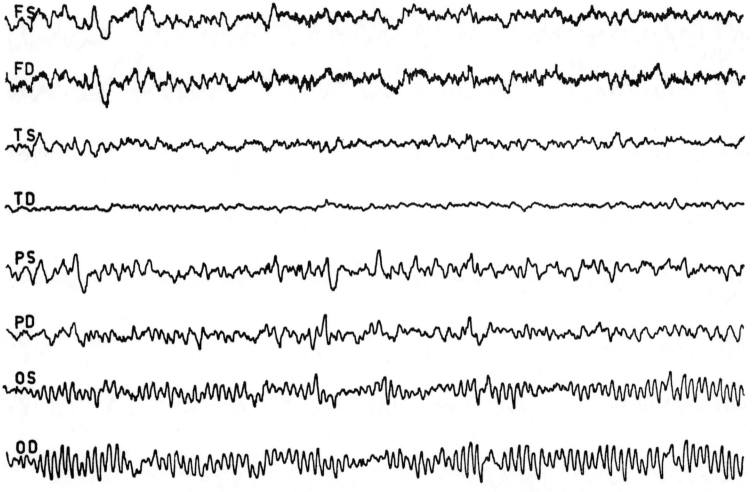

Regular, basic 9 to 11 per second sinusoidal activity in occipital leads.

FIGURE 68. — *Seven years, drowsy.* 91

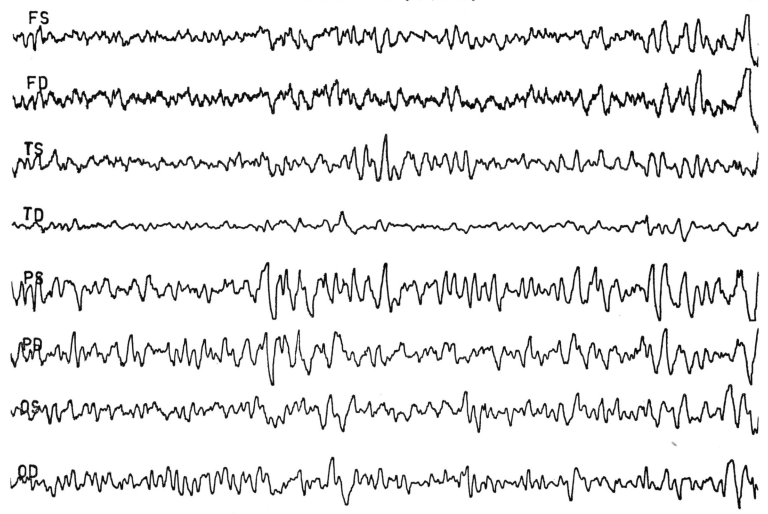

The transition from waking to drowsiness is characterized by a flattening of the occipital leads while humps have appeared in the parietal area.

FIGURE 69. — *Seven years, sleep.*

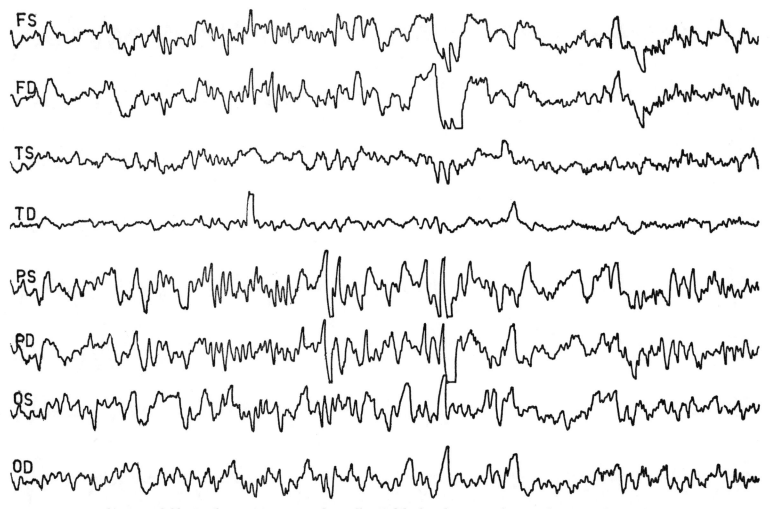

FS

FD

TS

TD

PS

PD

OS

OD

The same child. Twelve to 14 per second spindles and high voltage, synchronous humps. The artifact in the right temporal lead is a "pop" which is caused by poor contact of the electrode with the scalp.

FIGURE 70. — *Seven years, arousal.* 93

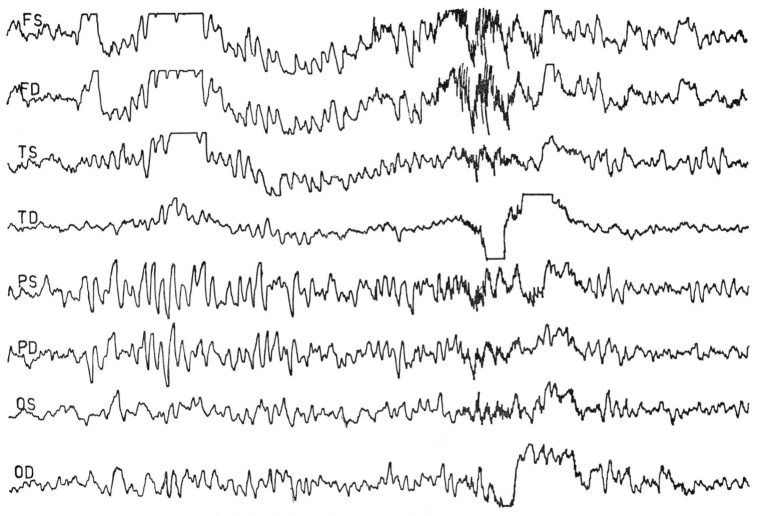

Some paroxysmal slowing in the parietal region with fast appearance of the waking pattern.

FIGURE 71. — *Eight and one-half years, awake.*

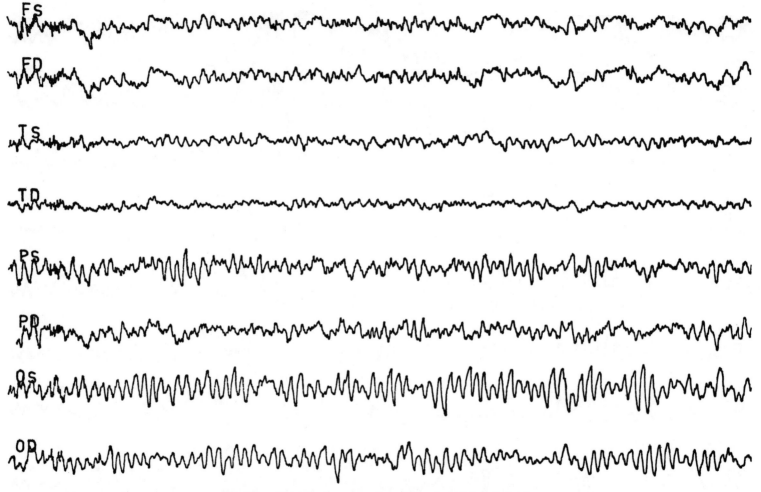

Regular, 6 to 9 per second activity in occipital leads.

FIGURE 72. — *Eight and one-half years, light sleep.* 95

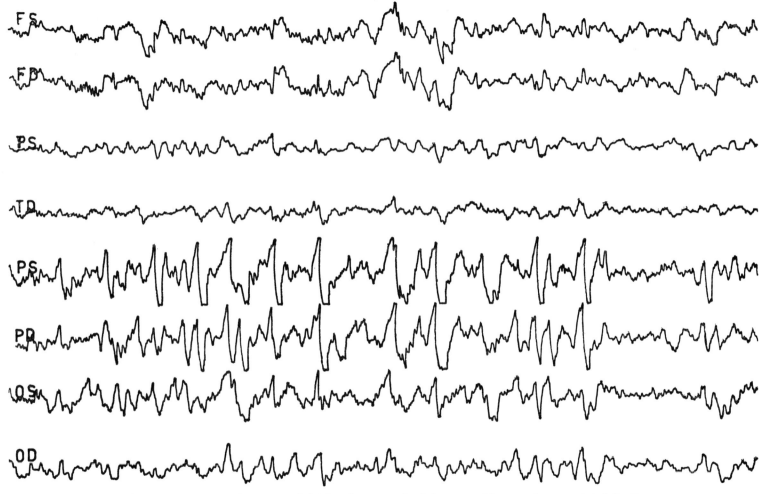

The same patient. A group of high, sharp, parietal humps with spread to occipital leads.

FIGURE 73. — *Eight and one-half years, sleep.*

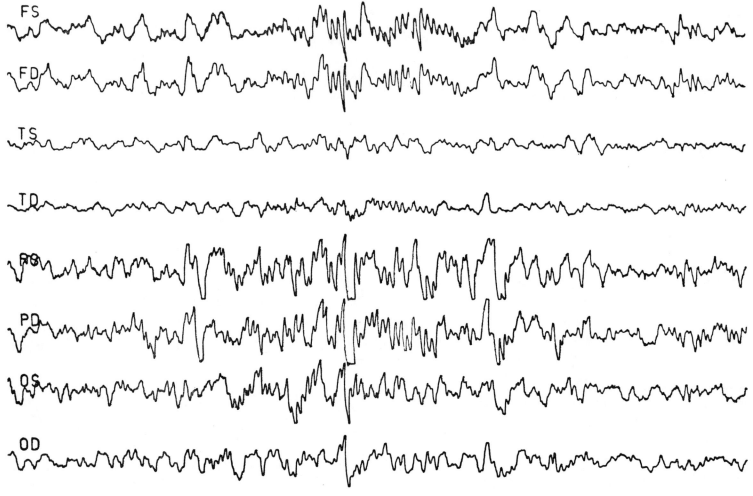

The same patient. Spindles visible in all leads, interrupted by high, synchronous humps.

FIGURE 74. — *Nine years, awake.* 97

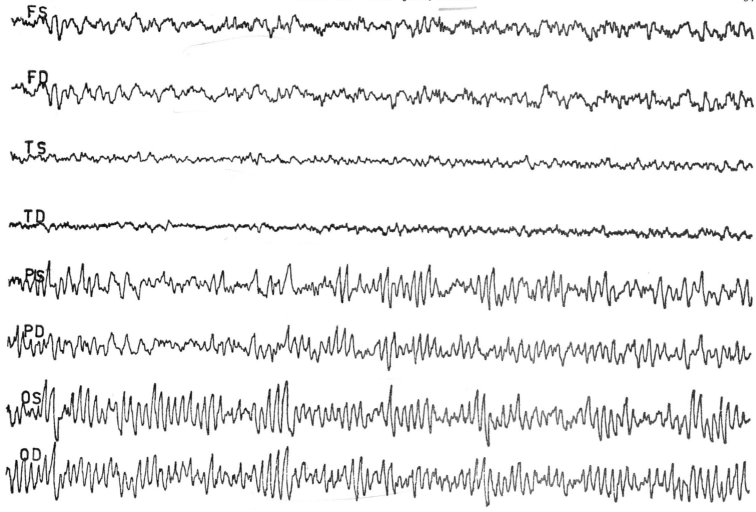

Basic 7 to 10 per second activity; the waves are rather sharp, a quality which is normal to about fifteen to eighteen years.

FIGURE 75. — *Nine years, drowsy.*

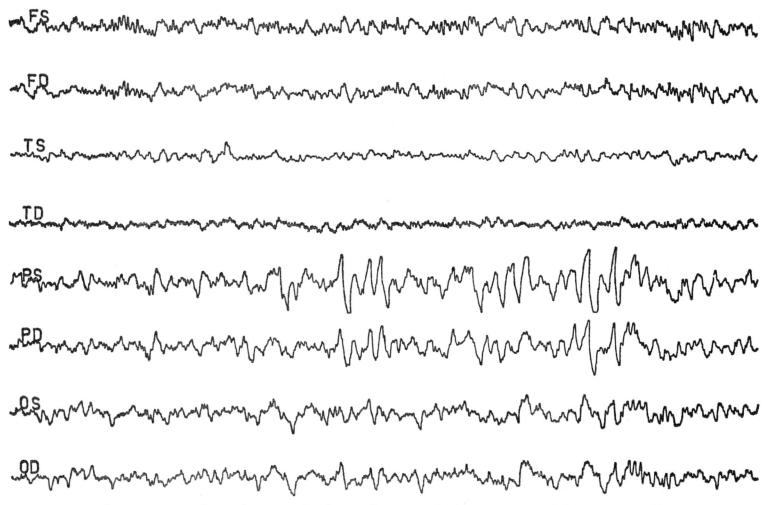

The same patient. Low voltage record with a small amount of 15 to 18 per second fast activity; sudden appearance of humps.

FIGURE 76. — *Nine years, very light sleep.* 99

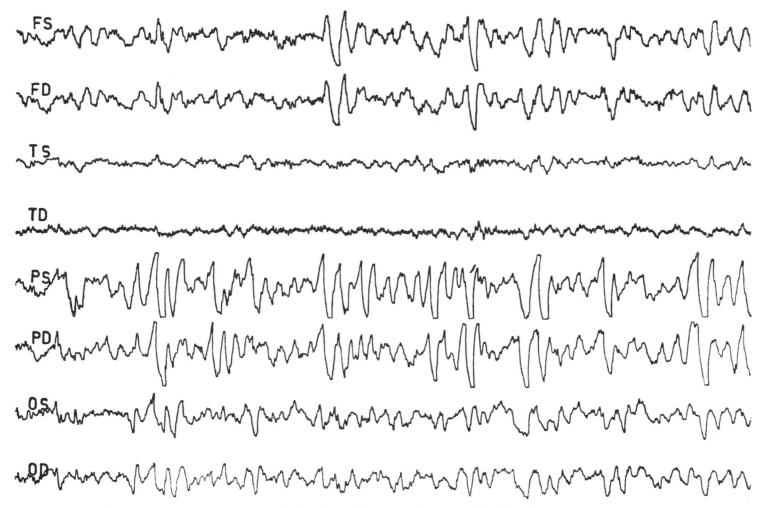

The same patient. Very many, high voltage humps in the parietal leads; also a few in frontal leads.

FIGURE 77. — *Nine years, sleep.*

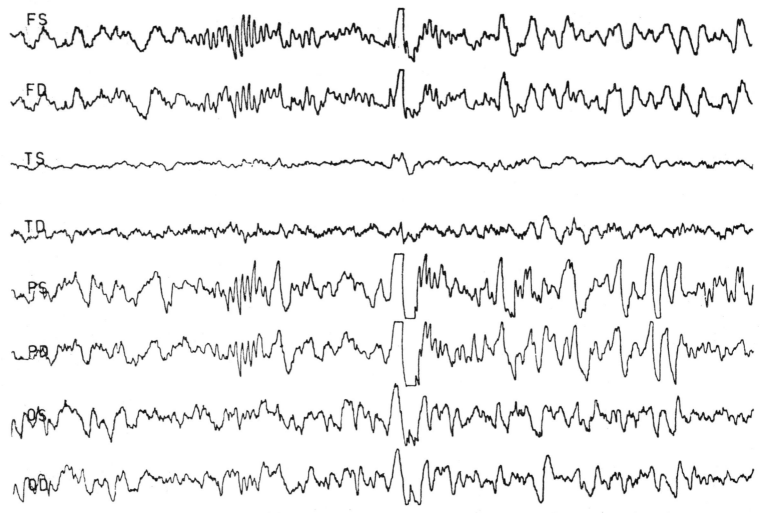

Humps and 12 to 14 per second spindles.

FIGURE 78. — *Nine years, very deep sleep.* 101

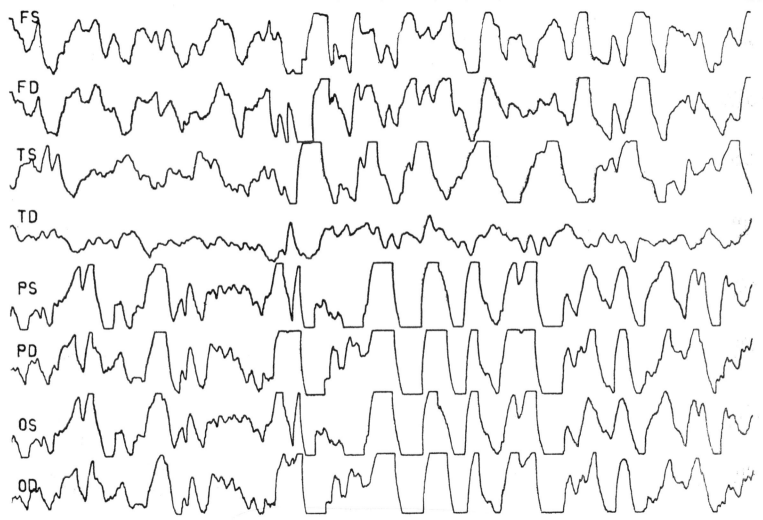

Very high, irregular, slow waves with frequencies of one-half to three per second in all leads.

FIGURE 79. — *Nine years, arousal.*

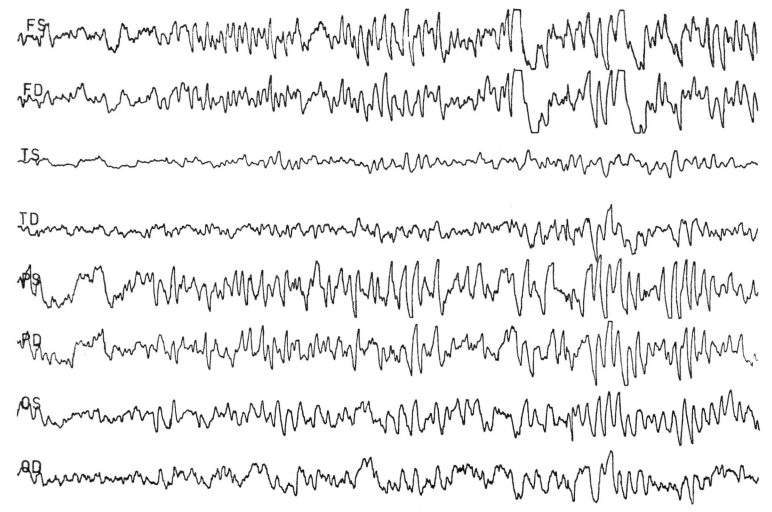

Paroxysmal 4 to 7 per second slowing; the very sharp waves in the frontal leads should not be mistaken for spikes.

FIGURE 80. — *Ten years, awake.* 103

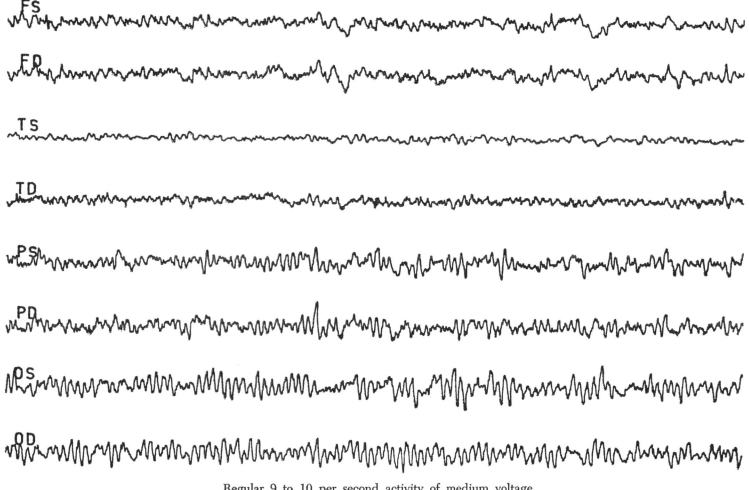

Regular 9 to 10 per second activity of medium voltage.

FIGURE 81. — *Ten years, drowsy.*

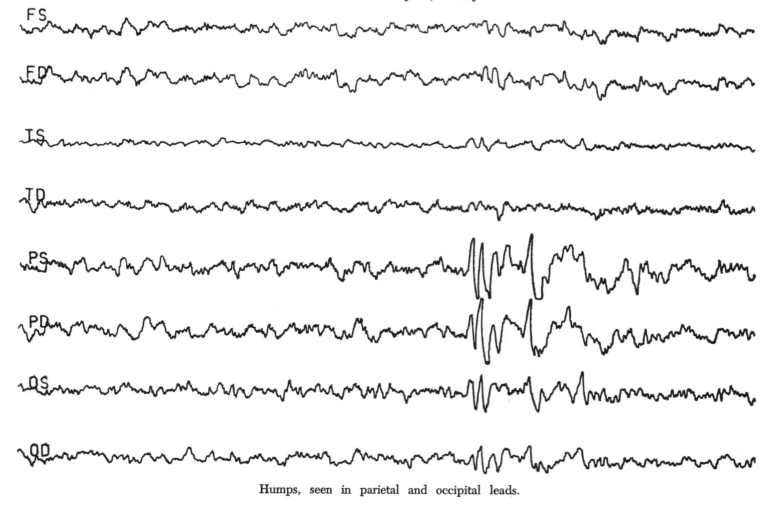

Humps, seen in parietal and occipital leads.

FIGURE 82. — *Ten years, sleep.* 105

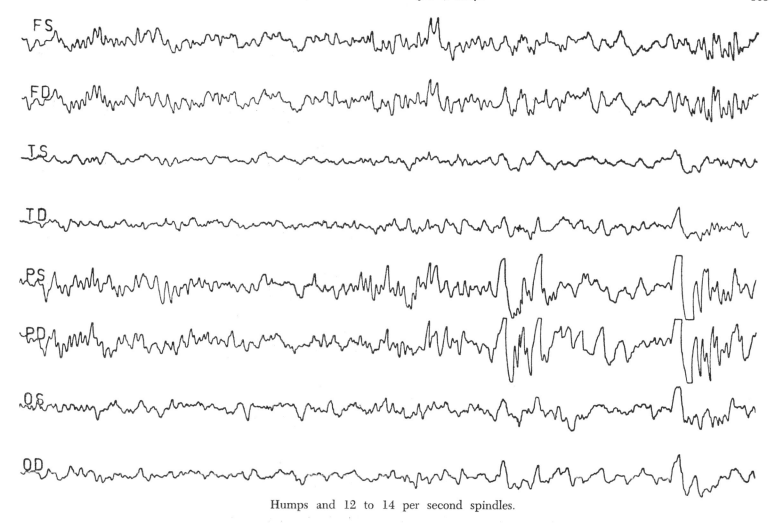

Humps and 12 to 14 per second spindles.

FIGURE 83. — *Ten years, deeper sleep.*

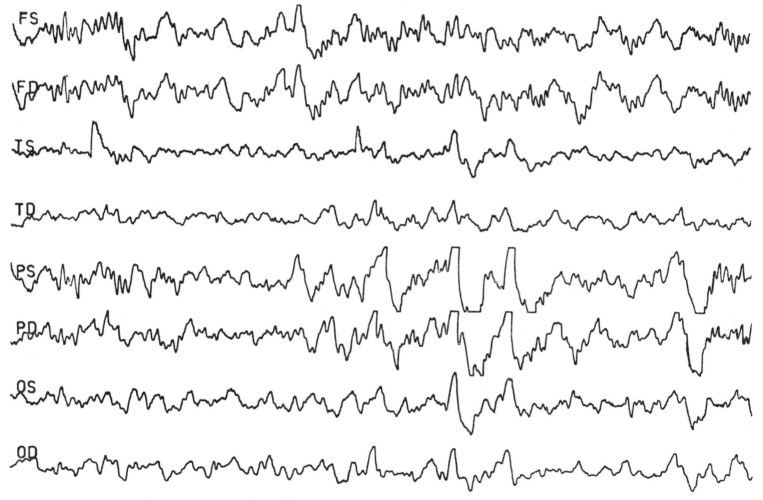

Ten to 12 per second spindles in frontal and parietal leads; "pops" in left temporal lead.

FIGURE 84. — *Ten years, arousal.* 107

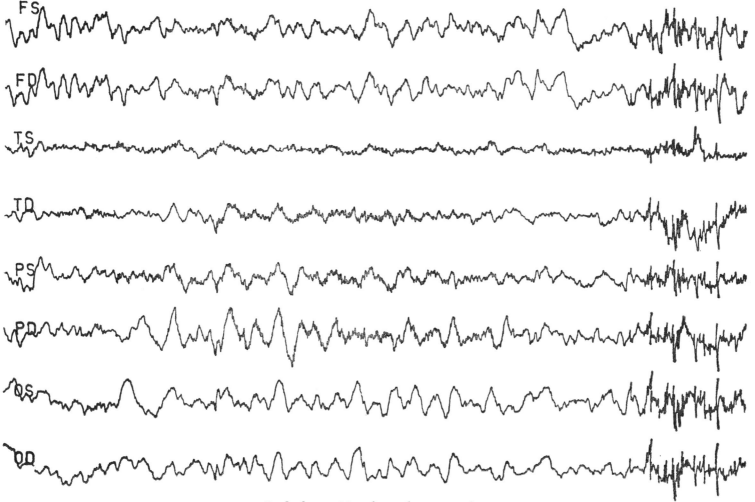

Gradual transition from sleep to waking.

FIGURE 85. — *Eleven years, awake.*

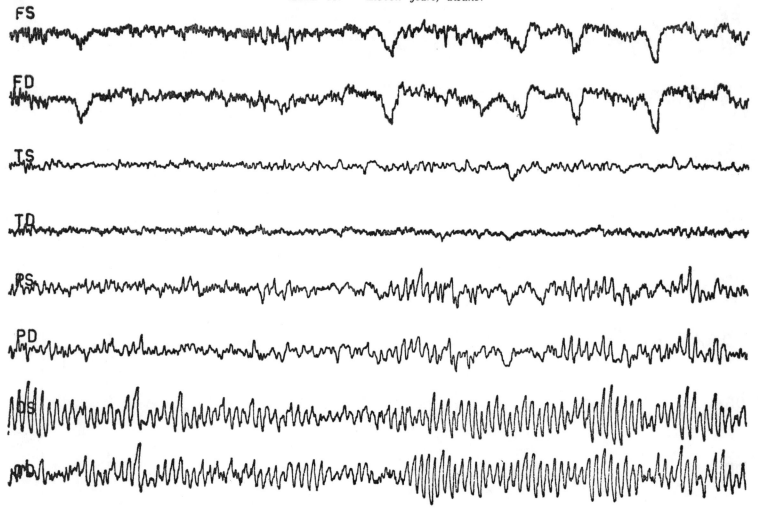

High voltage, 9 to 11 per second activity in occipital area.

FIGURE 86. — *Eleven years, very light sleep.* 109

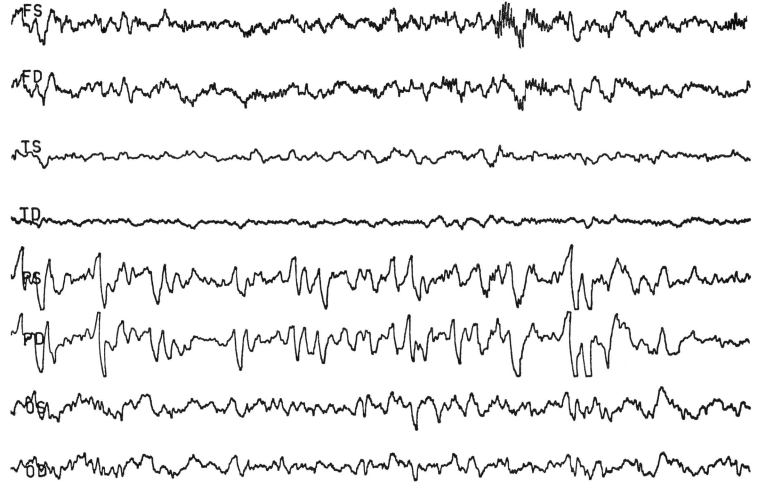

The same patient. Sleep induced by 80 mg. of Nembutal. Parietal humps and some 20 to 22 per second fast activity in frontal leads.

110

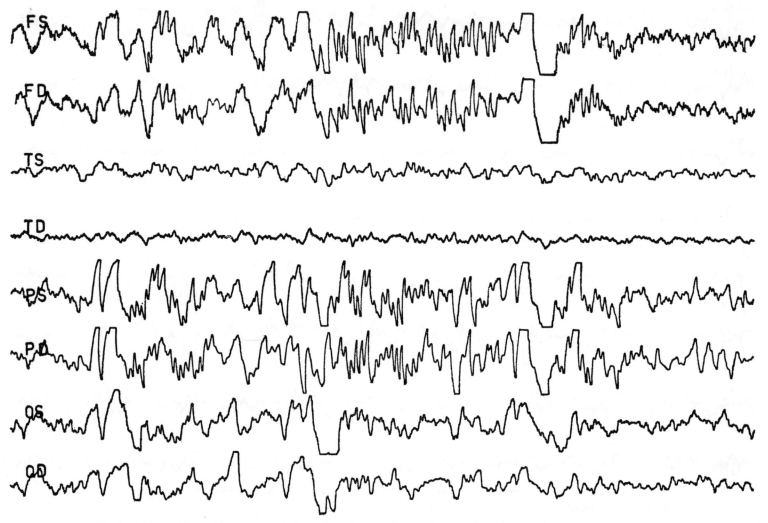

FIGURE 87. — *Eleven years, sleep.*

High voltage, 12 to 14 per second frontal and parietal spindles and regular, slow waves which simulate spike and wave discharges.

FIGURE 88. — *Eleven years, arousal.* 111

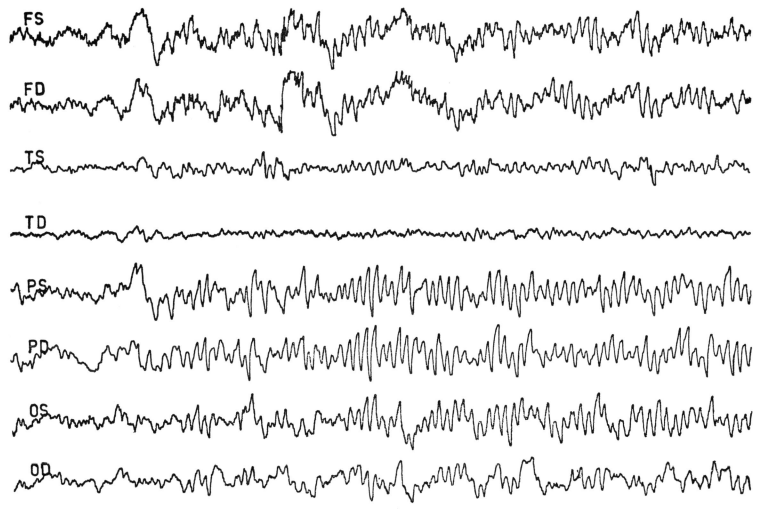

Sudden transition from sleep to waking without a special arousal pattern. Slight occipital slowing.

FIGURE 89. — *Twelve years, awake.*

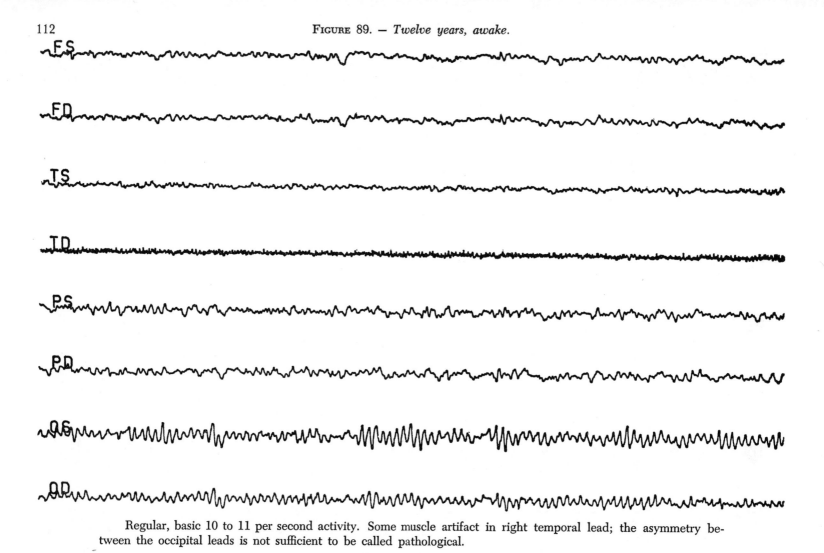

Regular, basic 10 to 11 per second activity. Some muscle artifact in right temporal lead; the asymmetry between the occipital leads is not sufficient to be called pathological.

FIGURE 90. — *Twelve years, light sleep.* 113

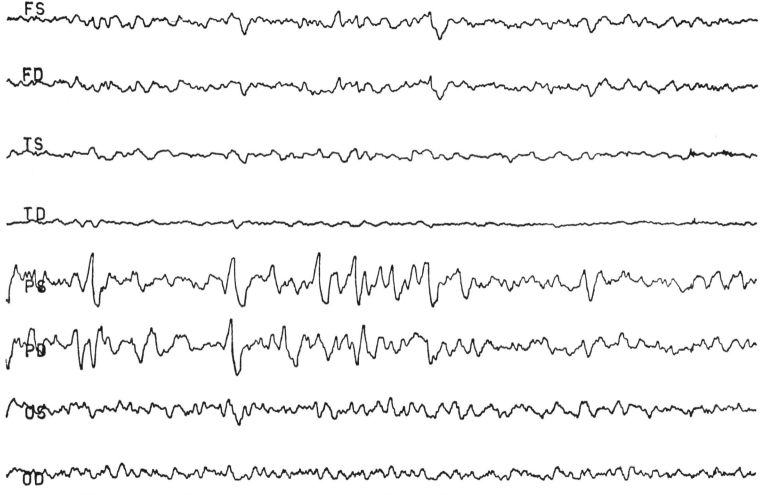

The same patient. The parietal humps are of a lower voltage now than they were in the five to ten year groups.

FIGURE 91. — *Twelve years, sleep.*

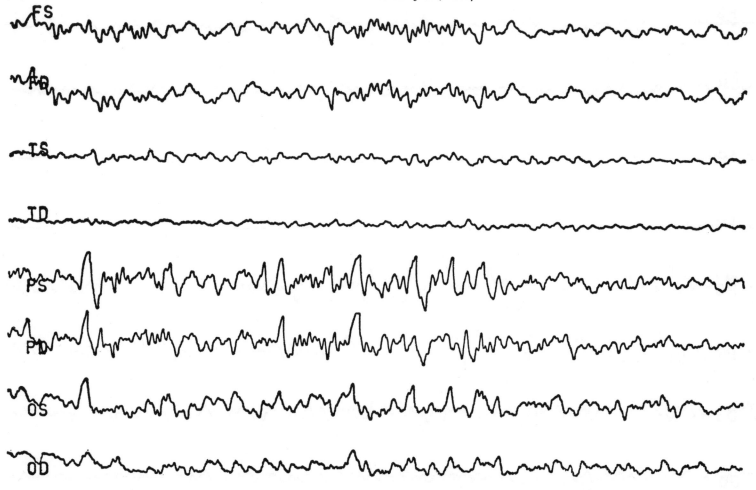

Humps and 14 per second spindles in parietal leads. Twelve per second frontal spindles are independent of the other.

FIGURE 92. — *Twelve years, arousal.* 115

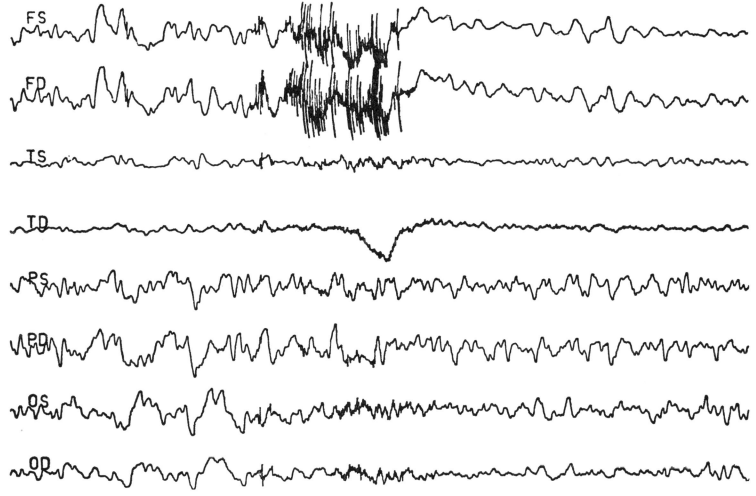

Less sudden transition compared to the previous illustration of arousal. Appearance of frontal muscle artifacts.

FIGURE 93. — *Thirteen years, awake.*

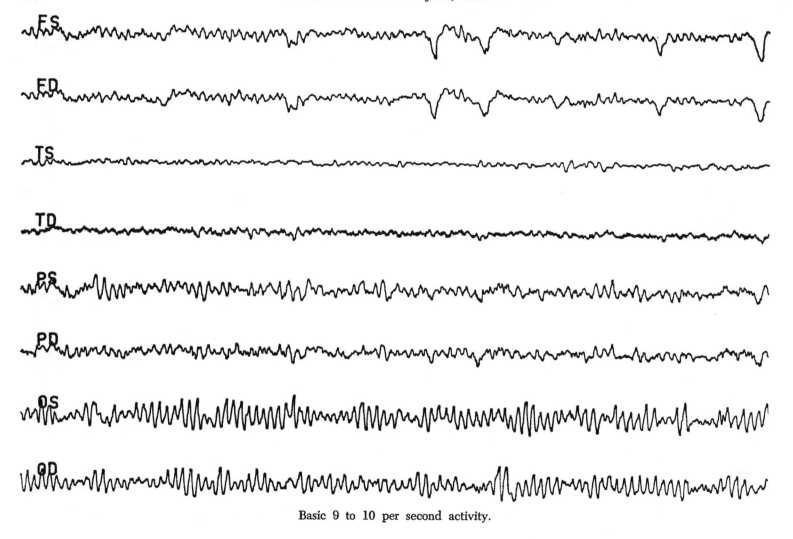

Basic 9 to 10 per second activity.

FIGURE 94. — *Thirteen years, drowsy.* 117

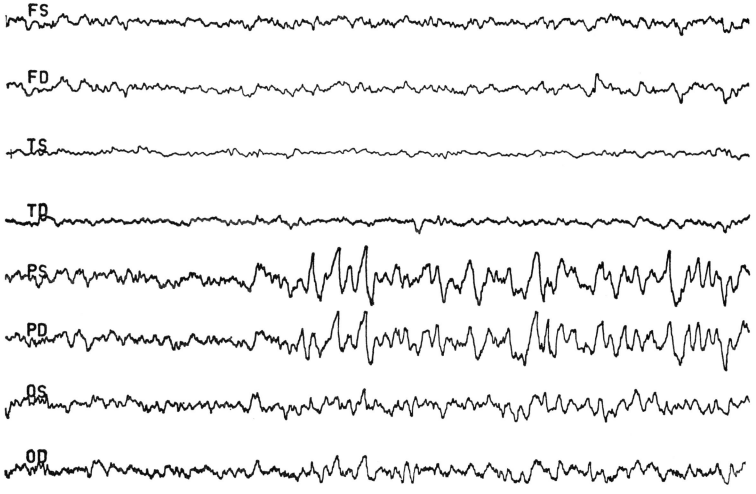

FS

FD

TS

TD

PS

PD

OS

OD

Transition from drowsiness to light sleep is marked by the appearance of parietal humps.

FIGURE 95. — *Thirteen years, sleep.*

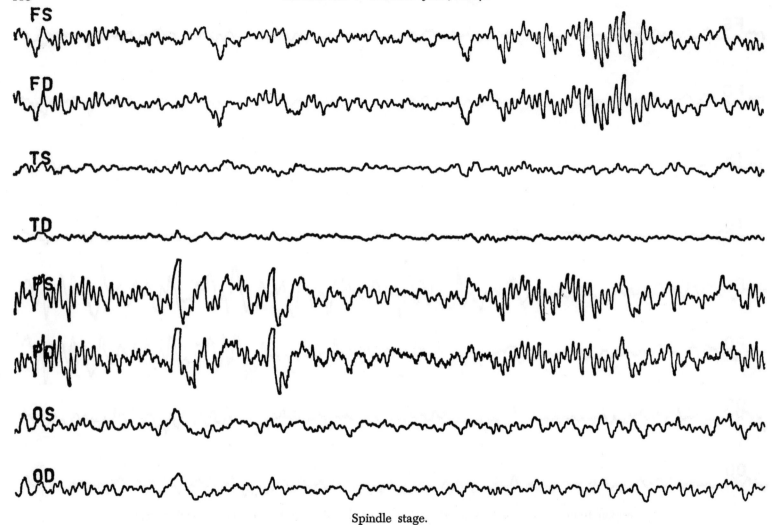

FS

FD

TS

TD

P'S

P'D

OS

OD

Spindle stage.

FIGURE 96. — *Thirteen years, deeper sleep.* 119

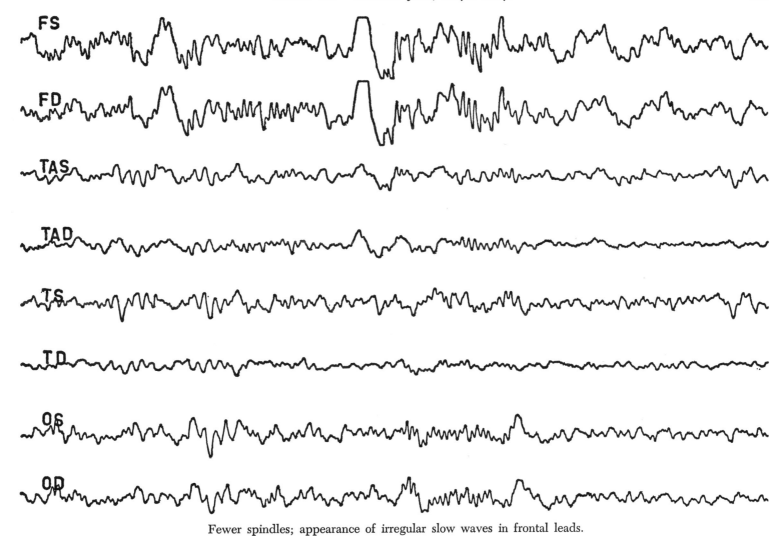

Fewer spindles; appearance of irregular slow waves in frontal leads.

FIGURE 97. — *Thirteen years, arousal.*

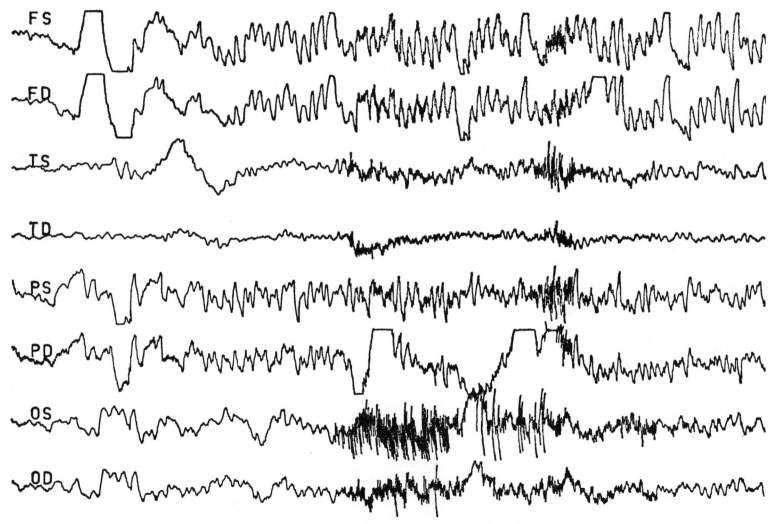

Runs of slow waves in frontal leads; much muscle artifact.

FIGURE 98. — *Fourteen years, awake.* 121

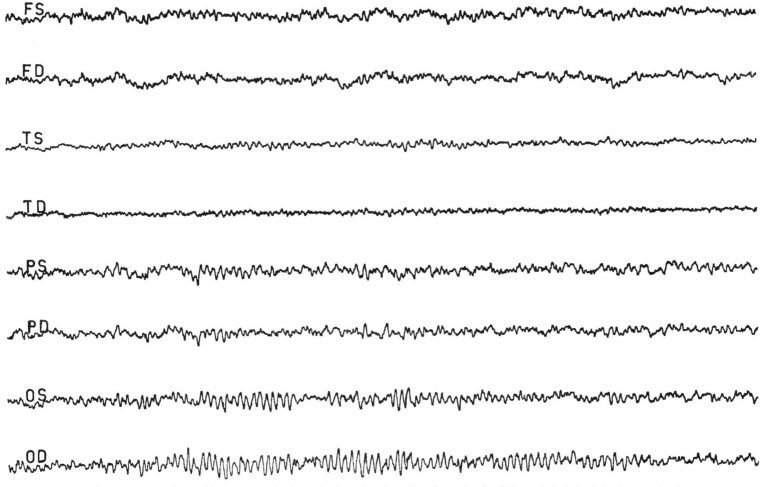

Basic activity 10 to 11 per second. The slight reduction of voltage in the left occipital lead is due to the beginning of drowsiness; at the end of illustration, the alpha rhythm is hardly visible anymore and the asymmetry has disappeared.

FIGURE 99. — *Fourteen years, light sleep.*

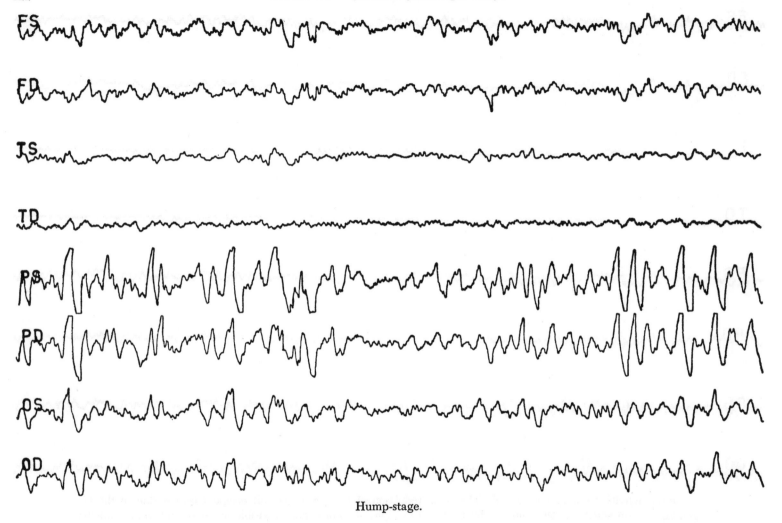

Hump-stage.

FIGURE 100. — *Fourteen years, deep sleep.* 123

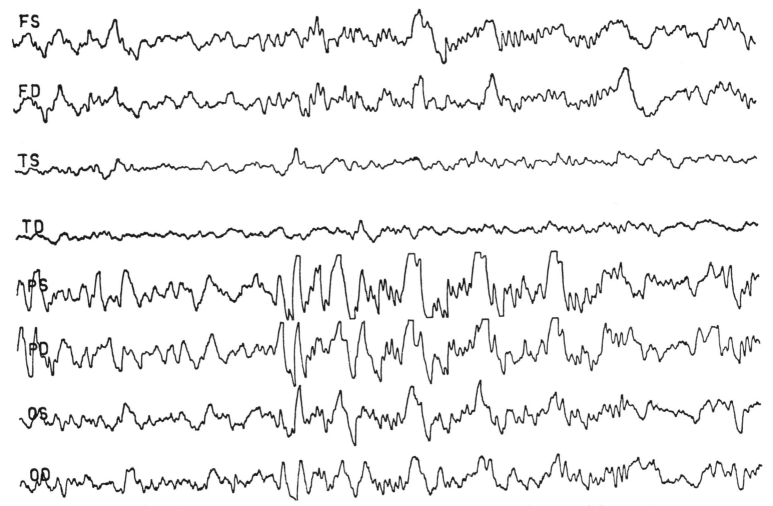

The spindles have a frequency of about 12 per second; the slow waves of this stage of sleep are in appearance similar to humps.

FIGURE 101. — *Fourteen years, arousal.*

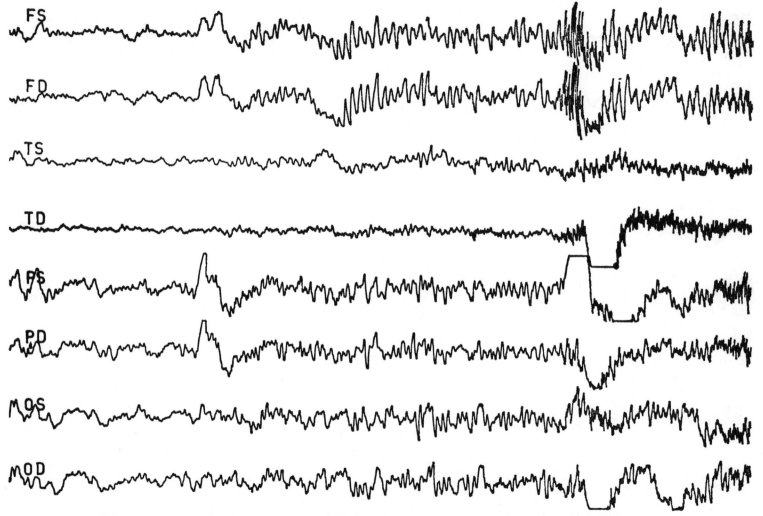

The same patient. A few 6 to 7 per second waves in frontal leads; 10 to 15 per second activity in all other leads. Appearance of muscle movement artifacts.